MIND-
BLOWING
SEX

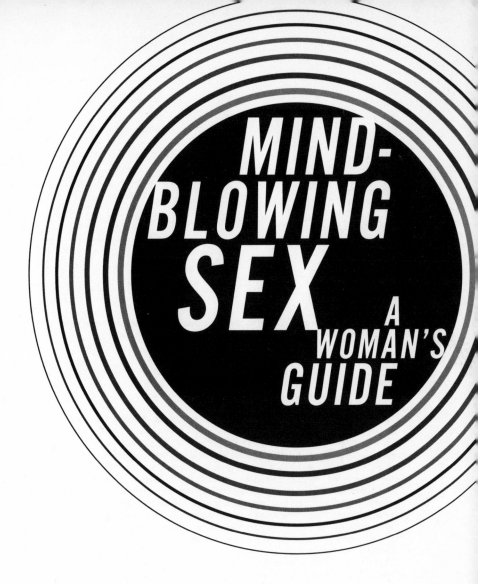

MIND-BLOWING SEX

A WOMAN'S GUIDE

Diana Cage

SEAL PRESS

Mind-Blowing Sex
A Woman's Guide

Copyright © 2012 by Diana Cage

Published by
Seal Press
A Member of the Perseus Books Group
1700 Fourth Street
Berkeley, California 94710

Library of Congress Cataloging-in-Publication Data

Cage, Diana.
  Mind-blowing sex : a woman's guide / Diana Cage.
      p. cm.
  Summary: "Confidence, health, and self-knowledge are the keys to a happier sex life—and sex expert Diana Cage is here to teach you how to achieve all three. *A Woman's Guide to Sexual Ecstasy* is an inclusive, hands-on guide to making sex more enjoyable for readers of all sexual orientations. Beginning with a brief historical overview, the book provides women and their lovers with an expansive view of female sexuality--from where it's been to where it's headed—and takes a contemporary approach to sex, offering direct tips and informed advice on how to have the best, most gratifying sex possible. Irreverent yet insightful, Cage covers both the emotional and physical aspects involved in increasing sexual pleasure—including tuning into your sexual fantasies, overcoming hang-ups, touching and being touched, choosing and introducing toys, and understanding female anatomy and orgasms. Straight-talking and non-judgmental, *A Woman's Guide to Sexual Ecstasy* will help women—straight and queer—to open their minds, reject stereotypes, educate themselves and their lovers, and learn how to enjoy sex more than ever before." —Provided by publisher.
  ISBN 978-1-58005-389-1 (pbk.)
  1. Sex instruction for women. 2. Sex instruction. I. Title.
  HQ46.C34 2012
  613.9'6--dc23
                              2011042048

9 8 7 6 5 4 3 2 1

Cover design by Kimberly Glyder
Interior design by meganjonesdesign.com

Printed in the United States of America
Distributed by Publishers Group West

FOR CHARLES

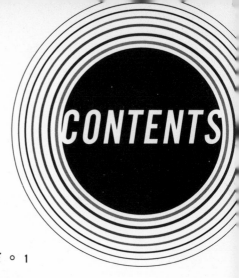

CONTENTS

INTRODUCTION:
WELCOME TO PARADISE

THIS IS A book about sex. It's also a book about women, our bodies, how we use them, how they work, and why they sometimes don't work the way we'd like them to. It's a book about sexuality, eroticism, pornography, desire, arousal, and satiation. Included in this book is only the tiniest bit of science, because I'm not a scientist. I'm a bit of a sexologist, if a sexologist is a person who studies sex. Truthfully, I'm more like a sexual adventurer, a sex writer, thinker, critic, and philosopher. Mostly I get called a sexpert, but I'm not sure anyone is ever an expert at sex.

This book is also about love, to a certain degree, in that loving oneself is a necessary component of mind-blowing sex.

Together we're going to take a tour of our bodies and our sexuality. Sexual shame often prevents us from really getting a good look at ourselves. There is plenty of talk about the wrongs of sex and the bad parts of sex, and yet there's very little information about empowering sex. Constant negative feedback about female sexuality affects our ability to explore our desire. Our sexuality is demeaned, trivialized, controlled. We're divided into categories like MILFs, Cougars, and Lolitas. So much meaning is attached to our bodies that there's barely any room left for any other expression of who we are beyond our physical selves. The female body is public domain. Our own bodies are used to sell us things so often that sometimes we forget we own them.

Something I know to be true, without a doubt, is that the more you understand yourself, the happier you are. This same concept applies to sex—the more you understand sex the better it is. And sex needs more attention from women—who are seen more often as sex objects than sexual beings. We need sex as much as we need food, water, shelter, and love. Great sex can be rejuvenating, healing, rewarding, and it can fulfill our deepest needs for intimacy and connection. Our desire to have sex with someone is how we know that a person is more than a friend. Great sex can make you fall in love.

When we feel confident, healthy, and sexy, our lives are happier places. Feeling sexy is like feeling invincible. But that feeling doesn't come easily in a society with a very narrow definition of sexy. Every outlet through which information can be disseminated will tell you what is and isn't sexy, but it's all misguided. Sex is personal; sexy is subjective. We can get turned on by anything and everything. Having mind-blowing sex is about rejecting the messages you receive about your sexuality that don't ring true to you. Feeling sexy and finding great sex is more about shutting out that erroneous information than listening to it. Once you've learned to navigate the perils of societal expectations and messages that keep you from fully being yourself, sex will become the most amazing, fulfilling, empowering experience you can have.

You may come across a new thing or two in these pages, especially once we get out of our heads and into our bodies. If you come across something unfamiliar, read about it. If it doesn't appeal to you, you don't have to do it. Don't be afraid of new ideas. Consider new paths to pleasure and don't judge paths chosen by others. At the very least you'll have some new topics with which to wow guests at your next dinner party.

I LOVE SEX. I especially love writing, talking, and reading about sex. I love kinky sex and vanilla sex, married sex, and casual sex. Rough sex, embarrassing sex, probably-shouldn't-have sex, funny sex, awkward sex, intimate sex, anonymous sex. The only bad sex is sex that makes you feel bad. Sex is liberating as long as we're liberated.

I've divided this book into three parts. Part 1 is the foundation you need to get the sex life you want. It's about changing your attitudes, unlearning obsessive and self-harming behaviors, and letting go of the hang-ups that do nothing but hold you back.

Part 2 will teach you how to do all sorts of things better: introduce you to new techniques and give you a greater understanding of just how smoothly the physical side of sex can work once you've mastered the skills.

Part 3 is for sexual adventurers. It's for the single folks who want to remain forever memorable to their lovers and the married couples that want to take their sex lives to a whole new realm of sexual experimentation. Part 3 is full of advice about the little extras and the kinky fun. It offers advice for a lifetime of fulfilling sex.

For the two hundred-plus pages, forget sexual orientation and sexual identity; we don't need them right now. If you are female, by biology or identity, this book is for you. Straight, gay, bisexual, lesbian, transgendered, bisexual, queer, mainstream, alternative, urban, suburban, polyamorous, married—we have similar sexual needs. Our specific tastes and preferred techniques might vary, but our sexual response and basic physical and psychological requirements are pretty much the same.

With that in mind, I've done my best to be inclusive. Sometimes I address women with male partners, sometimes it's about women with female partners, and within the categories of male and female I address a whole array of genders. Femaleness comes in many forms, not all of them feminine. My own sexuality has manifested in so many different ways that while I call myself a lesbian, I have been, at different times in my life, straight and married, straight, married, and bicurious, polyamorous, nonmonogamous, in an open marriage, bisexual and single, the straight partner of a transgendered man, and for the past ten years, a lesbian in relationships with women. Regardless of the sex or gender of my partner, my body always worked exactly the same way. My sexuality was never about who I was having sex with, it was about who I was when I was having sex.

Gender gets a lot of attention in this book as well. Talking and thinking about gender is important to every type of couple. It's easy to get hung up on masculinity and femininity in bed. We've burdened all sorts of fun sexual acts with gender hang-ups. And that's got to go. Gender and gender roles can make sex exciting; there's a sexual tension that stems from our differences. But there's a way to enjoy gender differences without being imprisoned by them.

Understanding gender and our expectations around it is an essential part of accepting ourselves and our partners. Women are expected to fall naturally into a more passive role in bed. It's something we're taught as children: women should wait around for someone to want them, for the man to ask them out and initiate sex. You might have desires that fall outside of traditional femininity but repress them thinking your partner won't find you attractive. Sometimes those of us who fall along the feminine side of the gender spectrum worry that our partners won't find us attractive if we aren't dressed up all the time. Or maybe we worry that the things that get us hot in bed will make us seem slutty or make us feel guilty. We sometimes hold ourselves back from real pleasure worrying that embracing what we want will make us seem less attractive.

These same insecurities affect our partners. Men, for instance, are often stuck in what they think is masculine behavior. And their fear of not being masculine enough prevents them from having all sorts of pleasure in bed that they could have if they let down their gender guard a bit. But it's not just men that are roped into this limited interpretation of masculinity, either. Anyone who identifies with masculinity can struggle with this. It's not uncommon for butch lesbians, transmen, or even women with masculine partners to quantify and qualify masculinity, policing it for transgressiveness and preventing themselves or their partners from experimenting sexually and socially.

If you are a man reading this book, or someone who identifies with a more masculine role, let me assure you that becoming a sexually realized, happy sex partner is about keeping yourself and your lovers from thinking too hard about right and wrong ways to express ourselves in bed. Anything—and I mean absolutely anything—fun that feels good to both of you is perfectly okay. Experiment with and enjoy the vessel you're in. There are so many ways to find pleasure in the body and you are only hurting yourself if you decide some are off limits.

I hope that regardless of who you are and who you sleep with you'll come away from reading this book with a new perspective, understanding, and acceptance of all the women around you.

I'VE WRITTEN THIS book for women because I am one. I know what it's like to move through this world as a woman. I know what it's like not only to have sex as a woman, but with a woman. And I know that our sexuality is still enigmatic, even to ourselves.

Chaucer wondered about what we really wanted when it came to sex all the way back in the fourteenth century. Freud wondered about it in the nineteenth century, and today so many researchers are still asking that question you could swing your handbag and hit one. Frankly, the question is dated and the answer is so obvious: We all want different things.

Simone de Beauvoir published *The Second Sex* in 1949. The "second sex" was women, she explained. The entire world was defined by men, and women were simply defined as "not men." All these years later this idea still shapes the way we see ourselves sexually. We're still struggling with what we want because female sexuality is simply defined as "not male." This is true whether you have male lovers or not. Lesbian sex is particularly mysterious for anyone who doesn't have it. "Which one is the guy?" everyone wonders. Or, if it is understood that there is no guy, the assumption is that it must not be "real sex."

Think of this book as a place where your sexuality exists outside of a partner. And if you can't picture what your sexuality looks like outside of a partner, then that's where you need to start: Figure out what it means for you to be sexual in a way that pleases no one but yourself. Together we're going to find new ways to be sexual and enjoy thrilling, liberating, mind-blowing, and life-affirming sex.

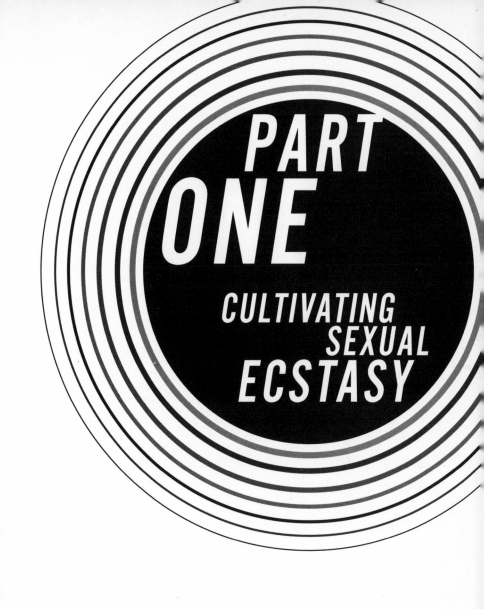

PART ONE

CULTIVATING SEXUAL ECSTASY

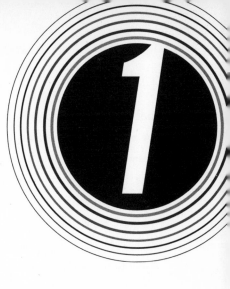

A SELECTIVE HISTORY OF FEMALE SEXUALITY

NE OF THE oldest and most famous depictions of the sexualized female body is the *Venus of Willendorf*. Dating back to 22,000 BCE, it's a limestone carving about four inches high of a naked woman with oversize breasts, hips, belly, and vulva, tiny little arms, and no feet. We don't know what she was designed for. Having no feet, she can't stand up, and she's not flat, so it doesn't seem like she's meant to be sitting on the prehistoric version of a knickknack shelf. She's carved from a type of limestone not local to the area she was discovered in, and, although no one is absolutely certain of her purpose, evidence suggests she was made to be held and carried around. The *Willendorf Venus* was the first of many similar statuettes to have been discovered; all are a similar size, and all feature prominent breasts, butts, and vulvas.

Scientists and art historians love to argue about the significance of these little statues, now called the Venus figurines, often with little evidence to support their theories. The generally accepted, mainstream interpretation is that they are fertility symbols of some sort—or at least that's what I learned in my college art history class, and I bet you did, too.

At some point in high school, I decided to rebel against my not particularly stringent, but still sort of Catholic, upbringing by proclaiming myself a pagan goddess-worshipper. This identity seemed very sexy and exotic, which suited my teenage self just fine. I read up on and adopted the myth of prehistoric matriarchal societies where fertility, childbearing, and the female body were revered. Some of this I took from two important books by archaeologist Marija Gimbutas, *The Language of the Goddess* and *The Civilization of the Goddess*. Being in high school, I wasn't exactly the most careful scholar and I'm sure I made up plenty of details on my own.

Somehow, the *Venus of Willendorf* figured prominently in my belief system. That little statue was, as far as I was concerned, proof that the patriarchy was a relatively modern invention, and that in prehistoric societies women were worshipped. It all sounded pretty good, and as an identity the goddess-worshipping thing went well with my penchant for flowy skirts and toe rings. Also, any time you want to make a case for mainstream beauty ideals being a creation of the mainstream media, you can point to the *Venus of Willendorf* and her nearly total roundness. Poor little Venus—everyone's got an opinion about her. The matriarchists claim she's a goddess, the art historians have suggested she's a fertility symbol, and some researchers have proposed that Venus is a product of women creating self-affirming representations of themselves, like an Ice Age *Vagina Monologues*.

So far, about two hundred Venus figurines have been discovered, all showing signs of having been handled and passed around. They were portable, exchangeable, and possibly collectible. The majority of them are naked, though a few are depicted wearing clothing of some sort, and a couple, found in the Russian site Kostenki, are wearing what look like restraints. As Timothy Taylor points out in *The Prehistory of Sex*, one figurine is wearing a breast-accentuating chest harness, and another seems to have her wrists bound together.

Given that these sculptures were dug up from the frozen tundra, it's not likely that a chest harness was functional clothing; it was probably just Stone Age lingerie. Which brings me to the disconcerting fact that, for all my early enthusiasm about ancient matriarchal culture, the *Venus of Willendorf* and the rest of the Venus figurines were probably just prehistoric pornography. Of all the theories out there, this is the one that the evidence actually points to. According to Cynthia Eller in *The Myth of Matriarchal Prehistory: Why an Invented Past Will Not Give Women a Future*, there's no more evidence for ancient matriarchy then there is for Santa Claus. I hate to admit it, but it looks like we've been seen as sex objects for two million years.

Fast-forward to about 3,000 BCE, when the Greeks were having sex all over the place. You'd think in a society rife with same-sex eroticism, women would enjoy a little more freedom, but you'd be wrong. Female sexuality existed (which is something, I guess), but it was thought to be very dangerous—a phenomenon that, if left unchecked, could cause women to tear men limb from limb in their quest to sate their unbridled lust.

Female lust, by the way, wasn't seen as a pleasure-based pursuit, the way men enjoyed sex; instead, women were thought to be driven by the reproductive function of the uterus. If not given what it wanted, which was pregnancy, the uterus would wander around the body, creating havoc and choking the life out of its owner. The Greeks kept the womb under control by promoting the necessity of marriage and childbearing. Women were called *gyne,* which meant "childbearer." They were considered property (a bit like cattle), were barely allowed to leave the house, and were valued mostly for reproduction. The Romans would divorce their wives for failing to bear children.

It got worse when the Christians showed up. The philosopher St. Augustine had a lot to say about women, and none of it was good. Augustine used to be somewhat of a wild man, having mistresses and indulging in various decadent pursuits, until he had a spiritual crisis that led to his converting to Christianity. Once he went religious, he became really down on sex. Apparently disgusted by his youthful escapades, he renounced sex completely, became celibate, and said everyone else should do the same.

Augustine promoted the idea that women were evil temptresses who would lead men astray and separate them from their rational minds. He was a very prolific writer and the author of over a hundred separate works on everything from Christian doctrine to incontinence. Propagated by word of mouth, his writings became accepted over time as the word of the church. Christian thinking had a rather lasting effect, and led to inventions like chastity belts that allowed men to lock up their wives, controlling their sexuality in a most literal sense.

Female sexuality took an odd turn in Victorian times, when the idea that it might be a normal function all but disappeared. The nineteenth century was harsh. The recommended treatments for the frightening, life-threatening diseases masturbation and nymphomania were generally application of leeches to the clitoris, vulva, and anus. Leeches were eventually replaced by clitoridectomy. Masturbation was thought to be life-threatening, that left unchecked it would lead to insomnia, exhaustion, neurasthenia, epilepsy, moral insanity, insanity, blindness, convulsions, melancholia, paralysis, and eventually coma and death. Women who had sexual feelings were subjected to elaborate medical treatments designed to dampen their desires, or were even committed to insane asylums.

Genital excitement led to hysteria and was believed to be caused by daydreaming and reading novels. The famed neurologist Jean-Martin Charcot believed that women's genitals were in fact the source of many diseases of the mind, including something called "menstrual madness." Charcot often held public tutorials on hysteria, attended by large groups of physicians. During these demonstrations, he would display the naked body of a female patient so doctors could inspect her genitals for signs of arousal and "illness." Famed psychoanalyst Sigmund Freud was a pupil of Charcot's and in attendance at these lectures, which puts some of his theories about female sexuality into perspective.

Upper-class Victorian women, on the other hand, were thought to be so chaste and sexless that men often visited prostitutes rather than subject their wives, bastions of morality that they were, to their base desires. So virtuous were Victorian women that their symptoms of sexual frustration were treated as something completely asexual. They were often diagnosed with hysteria and dispatched to physicians, who took care of their physical symptoms by masturbating them to orgasm in what seemed to be a very unsexy and routine medical procedure.

Hysteria, or chronic sexual frustration, as Rachel P. Maines explains it in her book *The Technology of Orgasm,* was the bread and butter of many physicians. It was chronic and incurable, and required regular office visits. The treatment for hysteria was an orgasm, which required a very hands-on approach by doctors. These arduous hand jobs often left the patients feeling much relieved, as you can imagine. Funny thing about all this: While we have to assume at least some patients were in the know, most sublimated their sexuality so successfully that these office visits were truly devoid of any risqué nature.

Prostitution was very popular in the nineteenth century, so much so that it sparked a sexual reform movement in New York and Boston as part of the larger movement toward social reform. Driven by middle-class white women, the sexual reform movement was a call for social morality, as well as for public heath, since syphilis was very common at the time. It was also spurred by racism and the "racial purity" concerns of white women who disapproved of their husbands' having sex with women of color.

In a battle that echoes today's ideological clashes between Second Wave and Third Wave feminism, middle-class white women wanted to get rid of sex work and teach sex workers domestic skills like sewing and cleaning. Sex workers, on the other hand, were resistant to forgoing relatively high-paying sex work for a hard living as low-paid domestic workers.

Social reform got more serious after the Civil War, and suffragists like Susan B. Anthony and Elizabeth Cady Stanton got involved. The social reform movement blocked a move to legalize prostitution in New York in 1867 and quickly spread to other sex-related issues, such as setting the age of consent and creating statutory-rape laws, sexually segregating prisons, outlawing abortion, opposing contraception, and censoring pornography.

In the early twentieth century, Sigmund Freud was in his heyday. To this day, you can blame him for nearly every annoying theory about female sexuality you've been subjected to, not to mention every orgasm you've ever faked. One of Freud's more famous and preposterous claims was that young girls suffered from penis envy. As you can imagine, this theory, which claims that little girls feel deficient because they lack the same organ that boys have, has gotten Freud a lot of play over the years, mostly because it's hilariously outrageous.

Freud also proposed the idea that having an orgasm through stimulation of the external head of the clit was immature and something girls would grow out of. A clitoral orgasm was an inferior one, and served as evidence that a woman had yet to reach full sexual maturity. A woman who really loved her husband was supposed to transfer her orgasmic feeling from the head of her clit to her vagina.

Margaret Sanger came along during the middle of the twentieth century. She started out as a nurse in New York, where she saw widespread misery among the poor, who had no way to control how many children they had. She realized the best way to help women who were stuck in this cycle of poverty was to teach them how to prevent unwanted pregnancies. In 1916, Sanger opened the first birth control clinic in the United States and was subsequently jailed for being a public nuisance and distributing obscene materials. Eventually, all the police actions against her drummed up public support and led to a 1936 court decision allowing doctors to prescribe contraceptives. Many states still prohibited the distribution of birth control, though; it wasn't until two U.S. Supreme Court decisions in 1965 and 1970 that the last restrictions were removed.

In 1953, Kinsey and colleagues rocked everyone's world by publishing the controversial *Sexual Behavior in the Human Female*. Though the book reported on myriad taboo subjects, such as orgasm, masturbation, premarital sex, and infidelity within marriage, most shocking to public sensibilities was the idea that women were as capable of enjoying sexual pleasure as men.

A little later, William Masters and Virginia Johnson published their groundbreaking work on the physiology of sexual arousal and intercourse. The sexual response cycle, as described by Masters and Johnson, begins with excitation, as blood rushes to the genitals in both sexes. Excitation is followed by the plateau stage, the state of arousal leading up to orgasm. After orgasm is the resolution phase, in which the genitals return to normal.

Their discoveries helped women, their partners, and medical practitioners understand the events of sexual excitement. They demystified the process of female genital arousal and lubrication, demonstrating that wetness came from the vaginal walls and not the cervix, as previously believed. They explained the physiological changes of the vulva, the engorgement, and hyperaemia. They detailed the changes the vagina goes through during different stages of arousal, including vaginal tenting during the plateau stage. And they explained the process of orgasm, which consists of involuntary contractions of the uterus.

In the 1970s, sex therapist and psychiatrist Helen Singer Kaplan added "desire" to Masters and Johnson's cycle. In Kaplan's model, desire comes first, then sexual excitement and eventually orgasm. Because desire is a psychological state, Kaplan's model emphasized the role of the mind in female sexual response and demonstrated the ways in which anxiety, fear, lack of communication, and lack of information can interrupt sexual response for women. Our understanding of female sexual response was augmented once again in the 1980s by gynecologist Rosemary Basson, who suggested that desire might lead to sexual stimulation, but sexual stimulation can also stoke desire. Basson's model more accurately explained female sexual response where desire often comes in response to sexual stimuli rather than spontaneously. Basson also asserted that orgasm did not have to be the only goal of sexual activity and that women could feel satisfied in any of the stages that lead to orgasm.

During the '70s and '80s, our understanding of the physiology of female sexuality was incrementally broadening, but society was determined to keep us in our place. A new wave of feminism, now commonly referred to as the second-wave, sought to raise our status in society by liberating us from oppressive gender roles. This was a hugely important time and laid the groundwork for the sexual freedoms we enjoy today. However, the sometimes-dogmatic approach taken by feminists in the '70s left some women feeling underserved by the very movement that sought to liberate them.

The feminist sex wars were a period in the '70s in which sexuality dominated much of the discussion about feminism. It started with concerns about lesbian sexuality and eventually grew into debates about all forms of sexuality, including heterosexuality, pornography, sadomasochism, butch/femme roles, and sex work. Pornography and its effects on the rights of women in society was quickly adopted as a main area of concern, and from this the antipornography feminist movement was born.

Very soon afterward, there was a backlash against antiporn thinking and the way it seemed tied up with negative views of sexuality in general. Some women, after fighting for so long to have their sexuality recognized, were hesitant to have it policed by well-meaning but strictly antiporn feminists. The two sides of the debate became polarized; tempers rose, debates ensued, and the sex wars were born.

The leader of the antiporn camp was a woman named Andrea Dworkin. Her rather extreme views—that pornography was responsible for every type of violence against women and that male sexuality was by nature aggressive and violent—were adopted as the basic rhetoric of the antiporn movement. In her book *Pornography: Men Possessing Women,* Dworkin asserted that the theme of all pornography was male domination of women, and that porn was thus extremely damaging not only to the women who performed it but to women everywhere, because men internalize its inherent misogyny.

The sex-positive camp believed that sexuality was a primarily physically pleasurable activity that extended beyond a simple need for bonding and intimacy for both men and women. Sex-positive feminists believed that a patriarchal society harmed everyone, not just women. This school of feminists was against censorship and suppression of pornography, explaining that these laws only served to further oppress sexual expression. An academic named Gayle Rubin was a prominent figure in sex-positive feminism; her essay "Thinking Sex: Notes for a Radical Theory of the Politics of Sexuality" is one of the theoretical cornerstones of the movement. In the essay, she calls for sexual liberation as a feminist goal and explains that we need to develop distinct theories of sexuality that are not just categorized under the umbrella of feminist thought.

Many issues raised during the sex wars still plague us today. Debates about pornography rage on, with some camps maintaining that it's an issue of violence against women and some claiming it's more a matter of free speech. Also hotly debated are questions about appropriate and politically correct sexuality. What's okay? What's not? Questions about the morality of rape fantasies, SM, gender roles, and virginity still loom large in public discourse.

Purity balls and virginity pledges, which promote sexual abstinence for young women, are yet another way in which female sexuality is controlled today. Among other religious-based debates about sexuality in the United States is the conversation about young people and sex education. Rather than offering comprehensive education about sex and sexuality, most schools in the United States endorse abstinence-only sex education, which promotes negative ideas about sex and strengthens the misguided notion that there are right and wrong ways to express sexuality.

While societal beliefs about our sexuality have been and remain complicated, a growing culture of sex-positivity has ushered in more freedom than we've ever before enjoyed. Today it's easy to find sexual information that places as much importance on women's sexual satisfaction as reproductive health. A new wave of pleasure activists and pro-sex feminists have joined the voices of sex-positive pioneers like Annie Sprinkle, Carol Queen, Barbara Carrellas, Tristan Taormino, Susie Bright, Nina Hartley, and so many others to change things permanently for the better. Despite the many obstacles we've faced, we continue to explore our sexuality, our individual turn-ons, and sexual wants and needs. When I look at today's sexual landscape, I see sexually empowered women everywhere I look. Sure we still have a lot of work to do, but we've finally reached a place where true sexual liberation is within our reach.

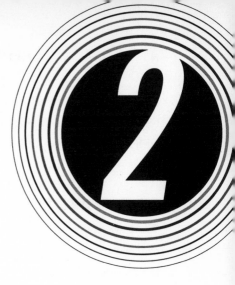

RETHINKING SEX

FEEL LIKE I'M always learning about sex. I read about it, write about it, talk about it at conferences, and, of course, have as much of it as I can, and I am constantly surprised by the amount of new information I encounter. Funny how much there is we don't know, when sex has been around as long as we have, and that's what? Four million years? Part of my job, as I've come to discover, is separating useful information from information that further obfuscates what we need to know to have fantastic sex lives. I enjoy thinking, talking, and writing about sex almost as much as I love having it. And not just the mechanics of sex—I also enjoy thinking, talking, and writing about sexuality, gender, culture, and society. I've spent my life combining those things. I know that my desire to understand who I am in this world as a woman and a sexual person, combined with my eagerness to master sexual techniques, is what makes me a good lover.

I believe that good sex requires an open mind, a willingness to listen and learn, and practical skills. This book is neither a thorough discussion of feminism nor an exhaustive list of bedroom skills. Instead, it's an introduction to the idea that the two things complement each other. Sex-positive feminism is something we're already familiar with. What I hope to provide you with is feminism-positive sex.

SEXUALITY IS CULTURE

What we think we understand about sex and sexuality has changed over time, and is still changing rapidly. Our sexuality is a cultural phenomenon, meaning that while our drive to have sex may be innate, the way we express ourselves sexually—for instance, the type of sex we desire, and what we consider erotic or taboo—changes based on the culture we live in. A lot of current thinking on sexuality still tells us that women are less sexual than men and are by nature heterosexual and monogamous. This thinking about female sexuality is rooted in a very sexist notion that females don't desire sex as much as men, and instead, being naturally powerless, use it as a form of currency.

For instance, many popular theories about female sexuality and infidelity purport that females, being less able to fend for themselves, have evolved to offer sex to multiple partners on the sly in exchange for things their partner can bring them, like food and protection. These are ideas we've constructed as a society because they reinforce the power of the dominant culture and have been upheld so strongly over time that they now seem as if they are part of our biological makeup.

We're in a period where it is very popular for science to link gender differences with biological differences in the brains of males and females. This is why contemporary sex and relationship advice centers on helping individuals understand "the opposite sex." Men are from Mars, women are from Venus, etc. We can't know for sure, though, that the development of our brains isn't somehow affected by our socialization as male or female. If the female brain is better designed for communication and empathy, as theories claim, and the male brain is designed more for linear thinking and spatial tasks, is it purely genetic, or is our brain development affected by our environment?

Contemporary theories about the biological differences between men and women, heterosexuals and homosexuals, are so easy to believe because they *seem true,* and backed up by *science.* Scientific discoveries, however, are limited by the way science is practiced, i.e., positivism, or the belief that knowledge isn't authentic unless it can be positively verified. This form of scientific inquiry favors the idea that all gender differences are biologically driven and innate, and that if we don't fit neatly into the prescribed roles that match our biological sex, then we are somehow deficient or, worse, deviant.

Science has offered misguided theories about female sexuality from the very beginning. Aristotle was sure that women were just men who had failed to grow penises in the womb. It was once thought that vaginas were penises turned inside out, that menstrual blood and breast milk were the same thing as semen, and that the uterus was simply a penis that had gotten stuck up inside the body.

The way we view sexuality and sexual practices is continually evolving, but not necessarily expanding and creating more space for sexual expression the way we need it to. Women with sexual urges are no longer diagnosed with nymphomania and hysteria, though sometimes I wonder if the prevalence of female sexual dysfunction diagnoses isn't just a repackaging of nineteenth-century disorders. Even beliefs about sex practices go in and out of fashion. The ancient Greeks practiced all varieties of homosexual sex, yet heterosexuality and homosexuality didn't exist the way we think of them now. Certainly, there was no hierarchy wherein one type of desire granted a citizen more rights than another. Today, we're so used to the idea that the world is split up into these two categories that it seems as if it must be dictated by biology. But heterosexuality and homosexuality as concepts have only been around for less than one hundred years. Before these terms existed, what you did in bed was simply an act, not the whole of your identity. Of course the shaping of sexual identities is an important part of understanding ourselves; however, it's important to note that the categorization of sexualities has also reinforced systems of inequality.

When we fail to look at the history of ideas about sex that came before us, it's easy to mistake current beliefs as part of some "natural order." But as Timothy Taylor points out in *The Prehistory of Sex: Four Million Years of Human Sexual Culture*, there is no such thing as a natural order. Ancient cultures hold vast evidence of human sexual variation, including homosexuality, transsexuality, transvestism, fetishism, sex as recreation, and sex as spirituality. Taylor also points out evidence that prehistoric societies practiced birth control and were fully capable of separating sex from reproduction. We created the rules, laws, and beliefs about sex under which we operate today. And since we created them, then it seems possible that we also have the power and perhaps even the responsibility to change them to make them more workable.

REVOLUTIONIZING SEX

Feminist philosopher Marilyn Frye noted that the word "virgin" didn't always refer to a woman who had never had sexual intercourse; it meant "a free woman, one not betrothed, not bound to, not possessed by any man. It meant a female who is sexually and hence socially her own person. In any version of patriarchy, there are no Virgins in this sense."

So, can a woman have complete agency over her sexuality in this culture that is, arguably, dominated by men? Feminists have asked this question for decades. I believe we absolutely can, but it requires us to fight against gender inequality, create more sexually egalitarian relationships, and risk disapproval from the less enlightened, which, let's face it, are the majority. The trickiest part is to find sexual equality without giving up the erotic excitement of power dynamics and gender. Creating egalitarian relationships doesn't mean we need to eschew masculinity or femininity. We want sexual agency, we want a great sex life, and we want to have these things while still being able to play with taboos, sexual domination and submission, and gender roles. I believe we can have all of that. In fact, I have found that the more liberated, knowledgeable, and sexually empowered I am, the more erotic charge power, taboos, and gender roles have in my life, precisely because I am not oppressed by them.

If you ask me, the sexual revolution is still in progress. It may have started in the '60s, but we've got a few more decades to go before we really let go of the last century or so of female sexual oppression and inequality. The '60s were a start, but we failed to uncover what we really wanted out of sex then. Birth control allowed us to have casual partners more easily, but it didn't make them more interesting or better in bed. The Pill didn't teach us about our sexual response or how to figure out what got us off, let alone talk about it. It was a bit like marching out of the sexual dark ages into a dimly lit room.

Because we had just come out of the nuclear-family model of the '50s, the '60s got us excited about the prospect of greater sexual freedom. Braless and hopeful, we set out to forge a new path. We wanted to find ourselves, but we had no idea where to look. We were still struggling to liberate ourselves from the only identities that we believed were available to us—wife, mother, and daughter. Several decades later, we've gone from no bras to push-up bras. We have careers, lives, high heels, and vibrators. We're liberated, we watch porn, we make out with strippers. Our friends are taking part-time gigs as dominatrixes to pay for their PhDs. So why is the sex still ho-hum almost half the time? We need a new model for sexual freedom, one in which our partners and the society we live in value our sexuality and satisfaction as much as we do.

SEX AND STEREOTYPES

In contemporary popular culture, sexuality is seemingly important only to the young, slim, white, and able-bodied. Images in mainstream media reinforce this idea over and over. "Woman" as a cultural category has a tremendous amount of things attached to it, especially when it comes to sex. Think about it: Women, as we define them presently, are passive and sexually receptive, unless they are manipulative and sexually voracious. Or they are hysterical, nymphomaniacs, or frigid, unless they are porn stars, sex kittens, virgins, and Lolitas. That's an awful lot of labels to navigate. And if you are a woman of color, sexuality is often convoluted by stereotypes about race. For instance, Asian American women are stereotyped as being sexually submissive and accommodating, while Latina women are often portrayed as spicy and hot-blooded. To be a sexual woman of color, you have to figure out how to get around the ramifications of being labeled "exotic" and "passionate."

For those of us who are not skinny, white, young, or exotic, there is no model of sexuality at all. We are assumed to be, or at least are portrayed as, sexless. This sort of cultural reinforcement makes it difficult to experience our sexuality in an autonomous way. What would female sexuality look like if we grew up away from media, away from messages about gender norms, racial stereotypes, and religious moralizing? I don't know the answer—do you? We have difficulty imagining what we actually desire because there are few visible options, other than those that exist to serve and reinforce the dominant culture. We have nothing to objectify but ourselves and other women. We've learned to love strip bars and girls gone wild because they all feed into our desire to be desired. But how do we experience and express desire for another?

Desire, sexual satisfaction, and orgasm truly are fraught more often for us than for men. It isn't because we are less sexual, dysfunctional, deviant, or frigid; it's because the ways we have been taught to fuck don't always serve our own sexual needs and desires. It's not that our sex lives are terrible—far from it! Most of us have great sex pretty often, and are willing to accept the not-so-great times as a normal part of having a sexual relationship. I believe, though, that we can make our sex lives even better and more satisfying by taking the time to learn and to teach our partners about our bodies and sexual responses.

Since ancient times, sexuality has been defined through an androcentric model, meaning that male sexuality is seen as the reality of sexuality, while female sexuality is deviant if it doesn't follow or complement a male pattern. With male sexuality at the center, expressions of female sexuality get labeled as pathological. For instance, the accepted model of sex—which includes desire, arousal, and orgasm, in that order—doesn't necessarily reflect women's experience. Sometimes we have desire but no arousal, or arousal but no desire, and we don't always end up with an orgasm. This gets us labeled as sexually dysfunctional.

In a widely publicized 1999 study of female sexuality, 43 percent of women ages eighteen to fifty-nine were described as having female sexual dysfunction, with "low desire" being the most common reason for the diagnosis. Forgive me for not being willing to believe that nearly half the female population is dysfunctional.

Men and women don't necessarily experience desire the same way. Social conditioning reinforces a model of male sexuality that assumes men are expected to have "innate sexual needs" and the desire to conquer a woman in order to get them met. The more sexual conquests he has, the more manly, dominant, and appropriately masculine a man is seen as being. Women, on the other hand, are taught to please while simultaneously being inundated with negative messages about sex. It's very convoluted. Women end up with a model of sexuality wherein they are allowed to be sexual only by male permission.

The androcentric sexual model has left female sexuality in a complicated place, and we haven't really had the time to figure out what we need and how to get it. But once we understand that there is no such thing as a "natural sexuality," then it becomes pretty clear that there is no reason why women wouldn't have their own sexual needs that look different from men's. I believe that once we change our thinking, we'll naturally change the way we have sex and re-create our sex lives in ways that better satisfy us.

RETHINKING DESIRE

As with arousal and orgasm, the common way we understand desire is modeled on male desire, and male desire is more often of the spontaneous variety: A man sees something he wants, gets a hard-on, and feels desire for sex. Additionally, a man's sensation of desire is reinforced by the visibility of his erection. Women's physical cues are easier to overlook, and studies show that even when we do experience physical signs of arousal, we still may not experience desire for sex.

Research sex therapist Rosemary Basson has proposed a new model for female desire, what she terms "responsive desire." While men may commonly experience desire in the form of spontaneous genital tension that they need to relieve, some women are more apt to experience desire related only to specific erotic stimuli. Many women who consider themselves sexually satisfied don't experience spontaneous desire in the form of genital tension, and without any erotic stimuli, they may not crave sex or masturbation very often. This doesn't necessarily mean that women crave sex less often, only that those of us who experience this responsive model of desire need to seek out erotic stimuli in order to get turned on.

Usually for us, sex is a conscious choice, and we seek arousal because we want to have sex, instead of seeking sex because we are suddenly aroused. We may decide to have sex because even if we aren't aroused in the moment, we know that once we get started, it's going to be great. Because the desire part doesn't come first, we create it by purposefully seeking out what we need in order to feel turned on. For some of us, that means looking at porn or reading erotica; for others, it means fantasizing. It could also mean getting ready for sex by masturbating, knowing that once we get started we'll become more aroused. Women who aren't experiencing desire as often as they'd like can learn to enhance their experience of desire by training themselves to trigger it by involving themselves in things that turn them on.

The most important thing is for us to take the reins of our own desire experience. It does us no good to wait passively for a partner to put us in the mood. The idea that we're all sleeping beauties waiting for someone to come awaken our desire with a kiss is a terrible trap. There is no way another person can know what we need to get turned on in any given moment. We can have better sex more often if we take control of getting turned on.

Keep your sex drive alive by engaging with erotic stimuli on your own terms, and then use the turned-on state you create on your own to have great sex with your lover. Keep some dirty books and a vibrator in your nightstand. Read some smut to get your juices flowing. Treat yourself to regular orgasms, whether you currently have a lover or not. Sex is a reward system—the more orgasms you have, the more you want.

Try this. List some past experiences where you found yourself really turned on seemingly out of the blue. What did it for you? A scene in a movie? A kiss? A fantasy? If you are in a low-sex-drive period and want to change it, it can help to think about times when you've really wanted it. Recalling moments when you've felt a rush of desire can help remind you that you do indeed enjoy sex, even if you are currently in a funk.

Write down five hot-for-it moments in the space below. Don't think too hard; just write down whatever comes to mind. You'll be jotting down notes quite a bit throughout this book. The process of writing helps you connect to your feelings. It also helps you remember things once you've brought them to mind.

1. _____

2. _____

3. _____

4. _____

5. _____

THE PERFECT SEX LIFE

Forget it. It's a myth. Buying into the idea that there even is such a thing is screwing up the sex life right in front of you. We're all convinced that somewhere out there people are having sex with easy-breezy, multiple, simultaneous orgasms every single time. That men have raging hard-ons that last all night; that women come from nothing more than vaginal penetration; that everyone has a perfect body, a perfect sexual response, nice, sweet, innocent turn-ons that don't make them feel ashamed, the perfect amount of intimacy, and uncomplicated feelings about love. The reality is, the couples who report the highest amount of sexual satisfaction are also the ones that have the most down-to-earth expectations and accept the limits of their bodies.

A 2006 study at the University of Arizona asked couples to record how they felt about each other every day for two months. Guess what? Even the happiest couples didn't always feel desire for each other. And some couples reported being hot for their partner one day and cold for them the next. The researchers also noted that couples who had the most positive feelings about their significant other overall were the ones who had the most passion for each other. The big passion-killers were negative emotions like anger, anxiety, neglect, and sadness. Buried anger and resentment toward a partner are sure sex-life killers. If you suffer from unresolved feelings, take steps to resolve them. They hurt you, they hurt your partner, and they hurt your sex life.

New-relationship energy, also called limerence, rarely lasts longer than three years. This is common and natural, and doesn't mean you've fallen out of love and your relationship is over. Rather, studies show that we get bored first. Once the new relationship energy drops off, we don't have the experience of spontaneous desire to fall back on, so we think we've lost interest in our partners and/or sex. The truth is, women who understand their sex drive and the sexual ebb and flow of relationship dynamics can re-create the early excitement phase. Sometimes it will be high and sometimes it will be low, but it won't disappear completely unless you let it.

Break your bad habits. Do you find yourself always saying no to sex because you think you are too tired? You might be tired, but that doesn't mean you can't get in the mood. Sometimes an orgasm is exactly the kind of relief a stressed-out woman needs. If getting turned on seems daunting, employ your vibrator to speed things along. Saying yes to sex can pay off by keeping us connected to our libido. Letting it go too long can make getting started seem even more difficult. So say yes to pleasure, even if it takes some work.

Explore new types of sex, and don't ever judge your desires. Female sexuality has been pathologized and stigmatized for too long. There is no such thing as "normal." It isn't any more normal to be straight, vanilla, and monogamous than it is to be into SM and anal sex. Get rid of rules and self-imposed restrictions. Do something new and maybe even kinky from time to time. Engage in sensual, sense-stimulating activities that make you feel sexy. Try limiting the major desire-killers—anxiety, worry, stress, fear—through self-care activities like yoga, massage, and talk therapy. Remember that you don't need a lover to be sexual. You can explore sexual stimuli like erotica and pornography regardless of whether or not you have a partner. Treat yourself to solo sex more often. Allowing yourself to be sexual and embracing your own desire outside of responding to a partner's needs is a major step in creating a more satisfying sex-life.

ALL ABOUT ORGASMS

3

W E HAVE SEX for many reasons, not all of them physical. But it's that mysterious buildup and subsequent release of tension called orgasm that keeps us coming back. I say "mysterious" because for women, orgasms are sometimes elusive. We can never be absolutely sure where our climaxes will come from, or if we'll come at all. Something that worked like a charm one week may fail us the next. Just as mysteriously, an unexpected erotic thought or passage in a book can work us into a froth, leaving us so aroused that an orgasm is only a few strokes away.

On average, an orgasm lasts anywhere from a few seconds up to maybe fifteen, though it's possible for a really big orgasm to last up to a minute. Some orgasms are all-encompassing; others barely register. Like anything else having to do with our sexual response, orgasms vary from woman to woman, day to day, sex act to sex act. It's perfectly normal to have off days, when even our tried-and-true methods for reaching that state of bliss will leave us wanting. And then there are days that surprise us, when an act we'd relegated to foreplay sends us crashing over the edge.

We can have orgasms from nearly any type of stimulation. Both Kinsey and Masters and Johnson have reported on women's having orgasms from nipple stimulation. Other sex researchers have described women's having orgasms from stimulation of the mouth and anus. Women have orgasms in dreams, and through fantasy. Women with spinal cord injuries have reported having orgasms through stimulation of their ears, nipples, breasts, and lips. In *The Happy Hooker,* sex worker Xavier Hollander's fascinating memoir, she describes having an orgasm from being touched on the shoulder by a cop. I myself once had an orgasm while reading an email! (At work, no less.) Granted, it was filthy and from a person I was head over heels in lust with, but still, I was so shocked I confessed to a coworker, who immediately replied, "I am never emailing you again."

Unlike men, women aren't held back by a refractory period. We're blessed with the ability to have as many orgasms as we want. As long as we continue to be stimulated, we can come, and come, and come again. Multiple orgasms are most likely when we remain aroused after we come, though many women find that their clitoris is hypersensitive after having an orgasm, and that indirect stimulation feels better than continuing to stimulate the clitoris directly. Try slowing down or stopping briefly before continuing stimulation.

TAKE THE PRESSURE OFF

An important note before getting into the hows and whys of women and orgasms: There's a sizable percentage of us for whom achieving orgasm is difficult; we rarely come during partner sex, if at all. If this describes you, don't waste your time feeling like a sexual failure. From time to time, orgasms are tricky for all of us. It's perfectly reasonable to enjoy sex without reaching any kind of *dénouement*; it still feels good both physically and intimately. Take the pressure to perform off yourself, and think of orgasms as a likely way to end sex, but not a necessary one. It's really no big deal if you sometimes don't come. It doesn't mean you are sexually inadequate; it doesn't mean anything other than what you make of it.

That said, if you don't come as often as you want to, keep reading for a discussion about making orgasms easier. Even if you come as often as you'd like, the same tricks that can make you come more easily can also help you to come more intensely.

When it comes to orgasms, the most important component is your mind-set. We hold ourselves back from pleasure in so many ways, so the first step in learning to come is unlearning the negative messages about sex and our bodies that hold us back from embracing pleasure. Start by convincing yourself of an obvious truth: It's not that you can't have an orgasm; it's just that you just haven't had one yet.

WHAT MAKES AN ORGASM

For the longest time, researchers were more interested in asking why we had orgasms than why our orgasms were difficult to come by. In other words, because female orgasms are not strictly a necessary component of reproduction, there's supposedly no real biological basis for their existence. Our orgasms are thought to be evolutionary leftovers, like male nipples. This is a stupid and troubling premise, of course. If we didn't have orgasms, if it weren't even an option, what interest would we have in sex? No real mystery there. There have been myriad theories about women's orgasms, from the (now discredited) "upsuck theory," which posits that orgasms help ensure conception by literally dipping the neck of the cervix into the pool of sperm and sucking sperm up into the uterus, to the idea that our orgasms and the resulting bonding hormones help us choose worthwhile partners with whom to raise children. It's my belief that knowing why we have orgasms is less useful for us than simply knowing that we are able to have lots of them, and that the more we learn about our sexual response, the more orgasms we will enjoy.

Beginning in the early 2000s, a new frontier of researchers have started studying orgasms in the lab, looking less for a why and more for a what and a how. Brain imaging studies show that orgasms are a mix of physical and psychological signals. It turns out that fifteen or so seconds of bliss have as much to do with your brain as they do with your bod.

WOMEN AND AROUSAL

Female sexual response is incredibly complex. One reason pharmaceutical companies have yet to come up with a satisfying female-centric substitute for Viagra has much to do with the way we experience the state of being "turned on."

In men, unless something is wrong, arousal leads to erection. Popular pharmaceutical treatments for erectile dysfunction work by relaxing the smooth muscle tissue that surrounds major arteries in the penis. This in turn allows more blood to flow to the penis, creating a firm erection. Erections provide visual feedback: A man looks down, sees that he has a hard-on, and thinks, *I want to have sex.*

For women, it's a more circuitous process. Even when our bodies exhibit signs of what would presumably be arousal—vasocongestion, engorged labia and clitoris, and vaginal lubrication—we may not actually be in the mood for sex. We need more than ready genitals to desire and go through with masturbation or intercourse.

One simple reason for the fact that we can be physically aroused but not desire sex or masturbation may be related to an inability to reach orgasm easily. An aroused man can stroke his erection or fuck his partner, and within a few minutes have climaxed, recovered, and put his pants back on. For women, that whole process is a bit more of a commitment.

Interestingly, Viagra has been show to have a similar effect on women as it does on men—namely, increasing blood flow to the genitals. However, while research has confirmed increased blood flow (through use of a monitor female subjects wore in their vaginas), that increased blood flow did not correlate with female test subjects' reporting that they wanted sex. In fact, in some cases women didn't register any sort of recognizable "turned on" feeling. They were often unaware that their vaginas were exhibiting typical signs of arousal. This tells us many things, but our main takeaway from this information should be that for women, wanting sex means more than being physically capable of having it.

Reading the medical literature and studying abstracts from clinical trials, we can easily see how little doctors and researchers understand about our sexual response. In one study I read, a doctor was quoted as saying, "Women who are not aroused can still perform." That sort of logic is very troubling. That doctor (and, I'm sure, many others like him) clearly equated "performing" with an ability to be penetrated, as if a woman's pleasure were completely insignificant.

In 2004, after nearly a decade of research and tests involving thousands of women, the makers of Viagra gave up testing the drug on women. It was finally understood that for women, arousal is a more complex process—it takes more than the simple ability to have sex to want it and enjoy it.

This whole idea works the same in reverse. It's possible for a woman to want sex and feel desire and yet not exhibit any physiological signs of arousal. This can certainly be frustrating, but it's normal. Unless you have trouble responding physically more often than not, and that interferes with your ability to enjoy sex, it's really not cause for alarm and doesn't call for medical intervention.

STAGES OF AROUSAL

That rushing feeling you get when you're fooling around is the result of blood heading to your pussy and pooling in your clitoris and labia. This pooling of blood causes those regions to swell. As more blood rushes to the region, your pussy lips plump up and your clitoris hardens. It also causes these regions of the body to feel warm to the touch and darken in color, and it gets the pussy wet by forcing moisture to seep out through the vaginal walls.

The clitoral glans grows longer and stiffer and pokes out from under the hood. The clitoral legs also stiffen and grow larger and longer, which in turn pushes out the inner and outer labia, making the entire vulva puffy and swollen. As you become more turned on, blood continues to flood the pelvic area, your breathing speeds up, your heart rate increases, and your nipples become erect. Your vagina responds as well, exhibiting changes in shape called tenting—the lower part of the vagina narrows while the upper part expands, making more room for a thrusting penis, fingers, or an object. If all goes well (i.e., the phone doesn't ring, your vibrator batteries don't give out, and your partner doesn't freak out or have an orgasm of his or her own), an incredible amount of nerve and muscle tension builds up in the genitals, pelvis, buttocks, and thighs—until your body involuntarily releases it all at once in a series of intensely pleasurable waves, a.k.a. your orgasm.

At the moment of orgasm, the uterus, vagina, and anus contract simultaneously at 0.8-second intervals. A small orgasm may consist of just a few contractions, while a big bang might trigger as many as fifteen. Other muscles in the body may also contract involuntarily; some women clench their fists or curl their toes. Women may vocalize, making grunting sounds or even screaming. Involuntary muscle contractions also account for the grimaces we make when we come. Your O-face is involuntary.

ORGASMIC CHEMICALS

During climax, the hypothalamus gives you a chemical rush of oxytocin. Sometimes referred to as the "cuddle hormone," oxytocin has been linked with bonding, feelings of affection, and the desire to protect one's partner. The same chemical triggers uterine contractions during childbirth and the milk letdown reflex in new moms. Generally, the more orgasms you have, the greater your bonding urge—this is one reason hot flings can be confusing. Have you ever blurted out, "I love you" after an orgasm? Blame the oxytocin. While you may have no intention of getting involved, have enough orgasmic romps with that sexy stranger, and your hormones may very well override your best intentions.

TYPES OF ORGASM

Your genital region contains a road map of sensory pathways, each path contributing a slightly different sensation to the feeling of orgasm. The three major players in our orgasmic response are the pelvic, hypogastric, and vagus nerves. The pelvic nerve transmits sensory information largely from the vagina and cervix, the hypogastric nerve transmits sensation from the cervix and uterus, and the vagus nerve carries information from the region of the cervix and uterus. We can experience orgasm triggered by stimulation of any or all of these nerve pathways, without any direct clitoral stimulation at all.

You've probably had the experience where an orgasm triggered by one type of stimulation felt different than an orgasm triggered by another type of stimulation. For instance, some women say that orgasms triggered by direct clitoral stimulation feel more intense and direct, while orgasms triggered by stimulation of the G-spot and cervix are more diffuse, with sensations spreading throughout the pelvic region.

A blended orgasm may very well be the best of all worlds. This type of orgasm is triggered by stimulation of multiple zones, each one carrying a different sensation and adding to the depth and complexity of orgasm. One researcher has nicknamed a type of blended orgasm a "trigasm," due to its being triggered by simultaneous stimulation of a woman's clitoris, G-spot, and anus. Labels are a fun gimmick, but you don't need to take them too seriously. Any type of stimulation that feels good and leads to a climax is successful. Don't worry too much about achieving someone else's orgasmic invention. Simply experimenting with your body and seeing what varied types of sensations you can trigger by stimulating multiple erogenous zones can lead to more fulfilling sexual experiences. We are all sexual explorers, so if you discover something great, go ahead and make up your own label for it.

ORGASM STALLERS

Why is it that some nights, no matter what you try, you just can't make it over the edge? Sometimes it's something simple: not enough direct stimulation, or stimulation that stops and starts, rather than sticking to a rhythm. In partner sex, it may be that our partners are anticipating our orgasms. In other words, you are getting closer, the tension is building, you've hit the stage where a climax feels inevitable, and your facial expression, breathing, and body movements transmit this information to your partner. Your partner gets excited and either quickens his or her pace in anticipation of your orgasm or possibly gets so excited from watching your enjoyment that it leads to having an orgasm of his or her own. While we all want our partners to come, that sort of thing can be a little frustrating if it consistently interrupts our ability to climax.

If this is something that happens to you on a regular basis, the easiest way to overcome this issue is to take charge of your own orgasms. Enjoy whatever it is the two of you like to do leading up to your orgasms, whether that activity is intercourse, oral sex, or something else, and when you get close, take over with your own hand or vibrator. Make it exciting for your partner by letting him or her watch while you put on a show and take yourself over the edge. That way, he or she gets to enjoy watching you in the throes of excitement, but you're in charge of your own pleasure, so the pressure is off and you won't have to worry that anything will go wrong.

GENETICS PLAY A ROLE

A 2005 study involving more than six thousand sets of twins indicates that the ease with which we reach orgasm is at least partly genetic. The majority of women surveyed reported reaching orgasm with varying degrees of difficulty, through varying methods. The results of this study suggest that there is no baseline "normal" when it comes to female sexual response, and undermine the notion that women who do not orgasm easily suffer from "female sexual dysfunction."

Difficulty with achieving orgasm is not at all unusual, and if our orgasmic response is at least partly dictated by our genes, it seems more productive to spend time finding new paths to orgasm that work on our individual bodies than to consistently feel disappointed when our bodies don't respond to something particular. If what you are doing doesn't work, it's not meant to be. Rather than feeling let down or wasting time doing the same thing over and over, why not scrap it and try something else?

Only a very small percentage of women surveyed reported never achieving orgasm at all, and because this study was self-reported—meaning, the women reporting simply filled out a questionnaire, with no researcher present to answer additional questions or clarify women's responses—it's probable that the subjects who reported not being able to orgasm had simply not yet learned how to do so.

THE PROBLEM WITH PERFORMING

Our resistance to letting go can also stall our orgasms. Have you ever found yourself feeling more like an observer of the sex you are having than a participant in it? Worrying about your appearance, your partner's enjoyment, and whether or not you are putting on a good show is a surefire way to kill your orgasm.

This behavior is really common, however. Observing, performing, third-eyeing, and generally thinking too much about what our partner is seeing, rather than giving ourselves over to the sensations of sexual pleasure, are all ways in which we sabotage our own sexual enjoyment. These are difficult habits to break, as we're so used to being sexually objectified that many of us internalize this way of seeing female sexuality. It feels very familiar to look at ourselves the way we want to be looked at. This leads us to compare ourselves to images we see around us, and if we don't measure up (and how can we?), we feel too inadequate to enjoy sex with the body we have. We're so bombarded with messages about our sexuality that ignoring them takes conscious unlearning—not something we're always capable of in the moment.

If this describes you, don't worry—you aren't alone. This behavior is reinforced everywhere; even well-meaning sex books aimed at women encourage behavior that takes us out of our bodies and puts us in a spectator role. It feels good to be desired, but being desired isn't enough to get us off. Through learning about our sexual bodies, we can learn to inhabit and own them. And hopefully, this knowledge will eventually lead us to sex lives so exciting that we won't have time to think about anything other than our own pleasure.

FOCUS, BREATHE, RELAX

The best way to prep for sex and increase your chances of climaxing is to engage in an activity that raises your level of arousal and decreases your stress levels. You have to relax to get off.

If possible, give yourself a transition period between your stressful day and the sex you are about to have. Try a presex bath or shower, especially a hot, steamy one with luxuriously scented body wash. Not only can a long bath or shower relax you, but intricate grooming rituals can make you feel sexy, confident about your body, and ready for sex.

Trading massages with your partner can also help; low-pressure sensual touching—or doing something else that feels good and connects you physically to your partner—can help ease you into a space where you can forget about your to-do list and feel ready for pleasure.

Masturbation is a nearly foolproof way to prepare for sex. If you are nervous that you won't become aroused as quickly as you'd like, presex masturbation can take some pressure off and allow you to focus on the good feelings sex is going to create. If you prefer to masturbate privately, try investing in a detachable showerhead. You can do double duty in your presex shower by getting clean and relaxed, and then turn the showerhead on your vulva and let the stimulating sensations get you ready for sex. It's okay to come this way if you'd like—remember, you can always come again.

If you are a braver sort, presex masturbation with your partner is a great way to make foreplay extra exciting. Let him or her watch as you touch your body with your hands or a vibrator. Your partner will find this very arousing, and you'll be in charge of your own pleasure. This is one surefire way to ensure you always get the amount of foreplay you need.

You may even find that your partner wants to masturbate, too. If so, great! The two of you can have an incredibly satisfying sexual experience together by simply masturbating to orgasm— no penetration necessary.

STAYING PRESENT

If you regularly have trouble coming, pay close attention to how much your mind is wandering next time you have sex. If your thoughts stray to worries about how long you are taking or whether or not your partner is bored, try working on staying present during sex. If you feel your mind wander to unhelpful thoughts, gently rein yourself in, pull your consciousness back into the present, and concentrate on the sensation of whatever activity you are engaging in at the moment. Literally concentrate on the minutiae of sensation. Focus in on the slightest motion: your partner's finger dragging across your clitoris; the toy, penis, dildo, or fingers stroking the walls of your vagina; the wetness and warmth of your partner's mouth.

Don't feel discouraged if you find that your mind wanders again after a few moments. Just bring yourself back every time. Keep doing this, and I promise you it will get easier. Staying present takes practice, but the payoff is an improved enjoyment of sex, as well as happier, more intimate relationships.

RETHINKING INTERCOURSE

On average, it takes women twenty minutes of direct stimulation to climax. It takes an average man less than five minutes. That's a pretty big discrepancy, wouldn't you say? These are just averages, of course; the amount of stimulation needed for orgasm differs from person to person. Still, these statistics apply to a sizable number of us.

If this discrepancy isn't an indication that penis-in-vagina thrusting isn't going to result in a satisfying sexual experience for both partners, then I can't image what is. P in V is fun, sure. It feels great. But it isn't the be-all and end-all of sex, and heading into it thinking of it as anything other than just one more fun component of sex is setting yourself up to fail. Most women do not have orgasms from intercourse alone. Our society's focus on simultaneous orgasm during intercourse is counterproductive. Not only is having an orgasm during intercourse not important to our enjoyment of sex, but our focus on it often prevents us from enjoying the many lovely orgasms we are able to achieve by other means.

Intercourse is awesome, but it's probably not going to lead to female orgasm. There, I said it.

GIVE YOURSELF A HAND

If you want to make intercourse more fun and maybe even come with your partner inside you, you'll need to find a position in which you can give yourself the extra clitoral stimulation you need.

Some women find that being on top works well for this. If you sit astride him, you have easy access to your clit and can control the angle of his thrusts as well. Some women are able to get the clitoral stimulation they need by leaning forward and rubbing their clitoris against their partner's abdomen while their partner's penis or dildo is inside them.

Something else to try is lying on your stomach with your hand beneath you so that you can rub your clitoris. Your partner can penetrate you from behind while you stimulate your clit with your fingers or a small vibrator.

We'll go into more depth about positions for intercourse in chapter 10.

SEXERCISING

Did you know exercise can help you have easier, faster, and stronger orgasms? While all exercise is good for your sexual health, exercising the muscles that surround your vagina and urethra can help your orgasms become more frequent and stronger. It makes sense, doesn't it? If the physical sensation of orgasm comes from a series of involuntary muscular contractions, then the stronger and healthier those muscles are, the stronger the sensation of contracting them will be.

The set of muscles that we want to focus on are called the pubococcygeus (PC) muscles. They were first discovered by a gynecologist named Dr. Arnold Kegel, which is why the exercises we do to strengthen our PC muscles are referred to mainly as Kegels. Dr. Kegel was simply looking for a way to help his patients with urinary incontinence, but as their bladder control improved, they also reported a fantastic side effect: improved orgasms!

You don't need special equipment to do Kegel exercises, though, if you want to get fancy about it, you can buy various objects designed to help you out, including barbells, insertable weights, and even gadgets that light up when you squeeze. We'll talk more about Kegels-ising contraptions when we discuss sex toys in chapter 11.

How to Exercise your PC Muscles

1. Pretend you're peeing. The muscles you are trying to locate are the same muscles you use to cut off the flow of urine when you pee. If you are very unfamiliar with this territory, you could try doing this exercise while urinating. Squeeze your muscles together to cut off the stream of pee. Got it?

2. Squeeze and release your muscles as many times as you can for one minute. Try varying the rhythm by squeezing and releasing in rapid bursts. Or squeeze and hold the tension for as long as you can. You can do these exercises anywhere—while reading this book, for instance!

3. Squeeze your butthole. Your sphincter muscle, or butthole, is the anterior portion of the PC loop. Follow the instructions above, only this time, squeeze and release your anus. You may notice that you carry a lot of tension in your butthole. Doing this exercise regularly can help you become more aware of the tension you carry and how to release it.

MOREGASMS, COREGASMS

Do you ever get turned on while you're working out? Do you know other women who do? I have a close friend who occasionally has orgasms while she's running. That's almost enough to make me want to go for a jog!

Turns out, it's not uncommon to feel sexual arousal and even have orgasms during strenuous exercise, especially during exercise that engages your abs and core muscles. For instance, I spent some time as a Bikram yoga fanatic and found that many of the poses I did in class would leave me feeling tingly. I never quite made it over the edge, but there were several times when I was pretty close—no easy feat in a 105-degree studio where everyone is sweating and the whole place smells like a locker room.

Bikram, like many other forms of yoga, requires a great deal of core strength. As you tighten your core muscles, you also build muscular tension in your pelvic area, especially in the PC muscles. As you tighten these muscles and tension builds, blood rushes to the area, creating the same pelvic congestion you get from being really turned on. The benefit from this type of exercise is cumulative, and building core strength improves sexual response like Kegel exercises do. Do it enough, and eventually you'll notice the difference in bed.

The exercise-induced-orgasm phenomenon is common enough to have been given a name: the coregasm. Women who report having coregasms say they most often come during very strenuous ab workouts. Do a quick Google search, and you'll even find suggestions for coregasm workouts. Hanging leg raises seem to be especially popular among coregasm devotees.

I've been on a quest to have a coregasm of my own, and while I've yet to experience it, I find the pelvic tension that builds up when I'm exercising to be very pleasurable, as is the idea that I'm in good sexual shape.

Coregasm Exercises

I asked a personal-trainer friend for some coregasm workout suggestions. While I can't promise these will get you off, they'll certainly help your sex life overall and are a nice addition to Kegel exercises.

THE BIG SQUEEZE

The first exercise—or sexercise, if you will—comes from yoga. This move is called a root lock. It consists of your curling up your pelvis, pulling your stomach in, and doing the hardest Kegel you can muster, all at the same time. It's more difficult than it sounds! Once you get the hang of it, try holding the squeeze for thirty seconds and repeat ten times.

The Plank

Another exercise designed to help core strength and possibly give you a coregasm is the plank. It's like doing a push-up, only once you are in the top of the push-up position, with your arms outstretched, you just hold yourself there for as long as you can. Twenty seconds into this one, you'll feel it in your abdomen and pelvic area.

The Boat

The final sexercise suggestion is another yoga move, called the boat. Lie on your back and raise your legs and torso up about forty-five degrees, so you are balancing on your butt and using your abdominal muscles to hold yourself up. Hold this pose as long as you can. Repeat ten times.

The one day I attempted all these exercises, I ended up being too tired for sex and had to just lie there while my partner performed oral sex on me, so I'd say my first foray into sexercising was a pretty great success overall!

ENERGY ORGASMS

Did you know some women can have orgasms without any sort of touch whatsoever? Author and sex pioneer Barbara Carrellas is one person famous for being able to do this, and has even demonstrated her ability to come this way on television a few times. If you want to know more about alternative ways to have an orgasm, I suggest reading Carrellas's amazing book *Urban Tantra: Sacred Sex for the Twenty-First Century,* in which she offers all sorts of explanations and instructions for non-genitally based orgasms.

How It Works

Sensation is energy. It's your brain sending signals from the body part being stimulated, and those signals get translated into the sensation of being touched. If we are touched in a way that feels sexually exciting, our brain sends signals to our genitals that we register as the feeling of being turned on.

We can stimulate feelings in our genitals by thinking about the feeling of being touched. In other words, we can stimulate our genitals with our brains.

So, how do you do it? Here are a few strategies to try:

1. Set aside plenty of time for this activity. And don't be disappointed if it doesn't work right away. Get yourself in a relaxed, happy, and sexy mood. Get rid of distractions, turn off the phone, etc.

2. Lie down. Get as relaxed as possible.

3. Imagine you can feel your clitoris becoming erect.
   Picture sensation in your genitals as a ball of tension.
   Use your imagination to heighten the feelings.

4. Fantasize. Fantasy can create real physical changes
   in your body. Fantasize about things that feel good.
   You can fantasize about an explicitly sexy occasion,
   another person, your lover, or simply the feelings
   in your pussy. Concentrate on feeling them build.
   Visualize the sensation. Give it a shape in your mind.
   Imagine it as a ball of energy you can move around.

5. Let muscular tension build throughout your body.
   The sexual tension that gets released during orgasm
   is actually real muscular tension, especially in your
   pelvic area. Try doing rhythmic Kegel exercises,
   slowly and deliberately squeezing your PC muscles
   and feeling that muscular tension increase.

6. Breathe. Our breath is linked to our arousal levels.
   Have you noticed that as you get closer to orgasm,
   you gasp and hold your breath? This is caused
   by involuntary contractions in your thoracic
   diaphragm, which is an arch of muscle under your
   rib cage that governs the expansion and contraction
   of your lungs. When it contracts, it flattens out,
   creating more space in the lungs so you inhale, and
   when it relaxes, it arches up, decreasing the volume
   of the lungs so you exhale. Tension and release in
   the thoracic diaphragm are like the tension and

release in your pelvic region. Conscious, rhythmic breathing will heighten your level of arousal. As you become aroused, you'll begin to breathe more deeply as your body's demand for oxygen increases, and then, as you get closer to orgasm, your breath will lock into this pattern. Pay attention to your breathing and allow it to change. Allow your arousal to grow with it.

7. Focus on the ball of energy in your genitals. Move it around rhythmically in time with your breath. Pay close attention. Let it build. Don't let your mind wander. Hold on to the tension long enough, and you may very well have an orgasmic release. If you don't, it certainly wouldn't hurt to give yourself a hand!

EMBRACING EROTICISM

W E GET THE concept of eroticism from the Greek myth of Eros. Eros was the god of love and sexual desire; he was known to the Romans as Cupid. Typically depicted as wreaking havoc with his pointed arrows—shooting them willy-nilly into unsuspecting bystanders—Eros was a mischievous little jerk. He loved to create as much drama as possible, which he did by wounding everyone unscrupulously—the catch being that some arrows caused their target to feel desire and some caused indifference. Thanks to Eros, everyone was always running around in some state of unrequited love—which was probably part of the reason the poet Sappho famously referred to him as bittersweet.

Eros as a concept is most easily explained as the drive for sexual and romantic love. The Greeks had a thought or two on the matter. The meaning and purpose of eros are the central subject of Plato's *Symposium*, his most famous play; each of seven characters gives a speech on the topic. Psychoanalysts (well, Freud) conflated eros with the concept of libido, or the drive to create life. The genius, albeit freaky, French writer Georges Bataille was obsessed with the erotic and described it as a psychological quest—a higher pursuit than simple sex.

EMBRACING THE EROTIC

We are all born with an innate capacity for sexual arousal and desire, which then gets shaped by messages we receive from the world around us—our upbringing, our lovers, social mores, literature, popular culture, everything. Our attitudes about sex and sexuality are a sum of all the experiences we've had leading up to any given moment. The combination of our innate sexual feelings and the cultural and emotional meanings we attach to those feelings is the foundation of our eroticism. By uncovering our basest desires, we can understand and embrace our erotic nature and thus expand our capacity for sexual pleasure.

What this means is that the most exciting part of sex isn't the physical process; it's the meaning we attach to the things we do. The meaning sex holds for us, the process by which we come to understand this meaning, and our feelings about what it means all make up our eroticism. Sex without eroticism is just an act or series of acts; it's just something our bodies can do. The erotic is how we feel about and experience our sexuality. Put another way, we can learn physical sexual skills, but without tapping into the erotic, we might as well be putting together IKEA furniture.

In his book *The Erotic Mind,* psychologist Jack Morin points out that eroticism is intertwined with all of our experiences, not just the positive ones. While sexual guilt, fear, and inhibition are bad for our sex lives, simply ridding ourselves of inhibition isn't going to automatically lead to amazing sex. Sometimes the things that make sex complicated—like guilt, anxiety, fear, and loss— also heighten its pleasure.

Take Eros and his arrows, for instance. No one got off scot-free; the targets who felt desire also felt the frustration of their desire not being returned. Sappho referred to Eros as bittersweet because she seemingly existed in a perpetual state of longing. In Sappho's poetry, the narrator often experiences intense desire yet is nearly always frustrated in some way. In "Fragment 31," one of Sappho's most famous poems, her narrator watches the object of her desire talk with another suitor. The poor narrator goes crazy, turns "greener than grass," and feels "Dead—or almost." Is she jealous? Well, we can't really know, but it sure as hell doesn't feel like simple jealousy. It's almost as if Sappho is eroticizing her own emotional pain. She finds it exciting to watch her love object talk to someone else. Her separation from her beloved inflames her passion. For her, the anxiety is erotic.

No book or expert can tell you exactly how to have great sex, because there's no one thing that makes sex exciting for everyone. A book can teach you skills, help open your mind, and, by normalizing sexual behavior, make you feel more comfortable expressing your sexuality, but until you tap into your eroticism and find your true turn-ons, you'll be largely going through the motions. Feelings are definitely sexual intensifiers, but that doesn't mean we have great sex only when we're head over heels in love. On the contrary, anything can trigger feelings that heighten our sexual experiences, not just love. Fear, anxiety, need, even ambivalence and indifference, can all be turn-ons. You may not find the sensation of yearning as exciting as Sappho did, but I assure you that you have some intense turn-ons, and getting in touch with them can take sex to a whole new level.

TUNING IN TO YOUR EROTICISM

The erotic is very personal—each individual has his or her own learned erotic attachments—and I can't tell you what yours are. I can, however, give you suggestions for discovering them on your own. I hope that by reading this chapter, you'll begin to think about things that may not have occurred to you before. As you uncover hidden motivations and learn new things about yourself, you may also find that your sense of self-esteem is heightened. Understanding your turn-ons and embracing them can give you a great sense of personal empowerment. I know it's possible to have life-changing discoveries about your sexuality throughout your life, because even though I spend all my time thinking, talking, and writing about sex, I still learn new things regularly.

CLEAR THE AIR

Ditch your judgments, both about yourself and about the people around you. Judging and fear of being judged take up too much space in our sex lives; plus, judgment ruins everything, and it's terribly boring. Forget what your mother told you. Forget what the neighbors think. Forget the sex-negative legislation that's constantly threatening to ruin your fun. For now, at least, we're going to put aside our feelings about right and wrong when it comes to sex.

We were all raised to think in terms of good and bad when it comes to sex, i.e.: Procreative sex = good; recreational sex = bad. Married sex = good; casual sex = bad. Thinking about romantic lovemaking = good; thinking about kinky, dirty, naughty things = bad. We could go on and on. This dichotomy is ubiquitous. For now, at least while you are exploring new ideas, let go of any good/bad categories. Let yourself go. Don't play thought police, and don't inhibit yourself.

Give yourself space to think about new things and new ways of being sexual. Why not? No one has to know. You're in the privacy of your own mind, and you don't actually have to go through with anything that doesn't sound appealing. Remember, thinking something is not the same as doing it. For example, I love scenes in porn and erotica with submissive females. I love having fantasies about being submissive, but I don't actually enjoy it in practice. I've tried it on many, many times, and more often than not, being in a submissive role leaves me feeling more frustrated than hot. I know it doesn't work for me in real life, and I'm fine with that, but I still enjoy the idea of submission and get a lot of pleasure from submissive fantasies. We all fantasize about things we wouldn't do in real life—that's what fantasies are for.

SEXUAL FLUIDITY

Labels help us define ourselves and are part of the way we interact with the world; however, they can also be limiting. Over the course of our lifetimes, we change and grow as individuals. It would be bizarre if we were the same person at forty-four as we were at twenty-four, yet it's common for people to define their sexual identity in their early twenties and never give it another thought. Viewing your sexuality as fluid can be a major step in finding and embracing your erotic self. There's no need to explain every time a shift takes place. You don't need to redefine yourself if, for instance, you have a same-sex fantasy or enjoy a different type of sexual experience. It's healthy and normal to try new things, to learn about ourselves, and to evolve.

WHAT'S YOUR SEXUAL PERSPECTIVE?

How do you feel about your sexuality and sex in general? It's a good idea to take time to reflect on this, because your attitude about sex is tied to your experience of it. Negative thoughts and emotions can surface during masturbation and partner sex and take away from our enjoyment. Your mental state and emotional health affect your libido, and a positive attitude about sexuality improves the quality of your sex life, making sex more fun, reducing guilt and anxiety, and making orgasm more likely. Your brain is your most important sex organ, so it makes sense to work on getting it primed for great sex.

One way to get in touch with your feelings about sex is to write things down. Journaling, making lists, and freewriting are great ways to tap into hidden feelings. Try something simple, like a list of sexual pros and cons, or make a "hot or not" list of various sexual activities. Let your imagination really run with this one—I mean, if you are going to do it, you might as well make it fun. Make multiple lists on multiple topics, if you like. Just don't email your lists to anyone! Once they're loose on the Internet, there's no getting them back. The general rule is: Never email anything you wouldn't feel comfortable having shown on *Entertainment Tonight.*

So, for example, my "hot or not" list would look like this:

Hot	Not
○ Outdoor sex	○ Whining
○ Kissing	○ Toe sucking
○ Fetishwear	○ Hairy backs
○ Lingerie	○ Tickling
○ Anal sex	○ Humiliation
○ Bondage	○ Scat play

HOT MEMORIES

Write down your ten hottest sexual memories. Don't be embarrassed—no one has to see this. Remember, don't judge yourself. Think about it: All over the country, conservative senators are running around in adult diapers, and if they aren't embarrassed, why would you be?

Just write down ten sexy memories from any point in your life:

1. _____

2. _____

3. _____

4. _____

5. _____

6. _____

7. _____

8. _____

9. _____

10. _____

Thinking about exciting previous sexual experiences will also help you have a positive view of sex, which in turn will lead to your feeling more sexual arousal and desire. Additionally, getting in touch with great sex you've had in the past can help you figure out what to add to the sex you're having in the present.

Once you've written down a series of memories, ask yourself: How do these memories make me feel? Are there any recurring themes? Any patterns? Was it fun to take a trip through my sexual history? What was going on for me during the period of time when I had these various sexual experiences? How do these experiences differ from the sex I am having now? Is there anything that went on in the above moments that I can re-create in the sex I am having now?

Now, make another list. This time, write down five things you find exciting that you have not yet tried.

1. _____

2. _____

3. _____

4. _____

5. _____

Sometimes just the act of thinking about new things helps us think positively about our sex lives. Reflecting on things we might like to try someday allows us to see our sexuality as full of untapped potential. Use your list of things to try as fodder for fantasy and masturbation, and see where it takes you.

CHEMISTRY AND EROTICISM

The current trend in the science of love and sex is to assign a biological imperative to everything we do. For instance, falling in love, and the subsequent focus and obsession we have on our love object, are said to be part of a biological drive that keeps us connected to an individual long enough to mate and raise offspring. The phenomenon of sexual chemistry also gets treated to a scientific theory—that being drawn to an individual you've just met is a sign of genetic compatibility. If you have "chemistry" with someone, it means that person is a suitable mate, and his or her genes plus your genes will make healthy offspring.

That's all fine and dandy, but I do think this explanation leaves out something obvious—our eroticism. Chemistry is more than a physiological response to the DNA information we gain through a partner's smell; sexual chemistry is also about the emotional response we have to someone who taps into our deep-seated erotic desires.

Look at it like this: If you find the idea of being saved exciting, then you'll probably go nuts if you meet a fireman. If you are secretly turned on by the thought of being in control, then a lover who waits on you hand and foot is likely to prove irresistible. More than being a reproductive impulse, the attraction between the person who wants to save and the person who needs saving is the psychological fulfillment of a symbiotic eroticism.

Leopold von Sacher-Masoch, the writer whose work gave us the term "masochism," describes his defining erotic experience in an essay titled "The Origins of Masochism." He traces the source of his obsession with submission to a beating he received at the hands of his haughty, fur-clad, adulterous aunt. She caught him spying on her while she was with a lover, and she whipped him to punish him. Sacher-Masoch was highly aroused by this experience, and from that moment on found himself sexually excited by glamorous, cruel, dominant women. Not all of us have something so easily traceable or so glamorously perverse, but hey, a girl can dream!

THINK SEXY THOUGHTS

A study by researchers at Grenada University showed an important correlation between the amount of sexual fantasies we engage in and our experience of arousal and desire. They concluded that having sexual fantasies gives us a positive attitude about sex and increases the amount of sexual desire we feel. In other words, if you want to feel sexier and have more sex, you can start by having sexual fantasies.

I'd like to encourage you to go wild in your fantasy life. In all my time as a sex writer and explorer, the people I've known who had the most ecstatic sex lives weren't the richest, smartest, or most physically beautiful—they were the ones who spent the most time thinking and talking about sex. There's a direct correlation between a positive view of sex, a rich fantasy life, and the enjoyment a person gets out of sex. Develop a richly erotic fantasy life and open your mind to new sexual experiences, and you'll find plenty of sexual ecstasy.

FANTASIZING IS NOT CHEATING

Some women worry that fantasizing about sex outside of their relationships means they aren't really in love with their partner or that their partner isn't "enough" for them. Nonsense. For one thing, having sexual fantasies leads to more sexual satisfaction, something that benefits your partner as well as you. Your fantasies are your own private cache of sexual thoughts that you can call on whenever you like. They are an important part of arousal and orgasm, and they enable you to be sexually self-sufficient, which in turn leads to greater satisfaction in relationships. Everyone fantasizes—it's a perfectly normal, common aspect of our sexuality. Studies show that 85 percent of women have sexual fantasies during partner sex. Sometimes we worry that fantasies are actually messages about unspoken and unmet needs, but this just isn't true. Fantasizing is about playing with ideas. Whether it's daydreams you have at work or fantasies you call on when you are about to reach orgasm, fantasies are part of being sexual.

EXPLORING EROTICA

If you need a little inspiration, try exploring erotica and pornography to get your sexual imagination flowing. I find that reading erotica or watching porn helps me to get into a sexy mind-set when I might otherwise be too overwhelmed by my busy life to engage in a spontaneous fantasy. Reading erotica takes me out of my day and transports me to a much sexier place, and once I'm turned on, I often find that my imagination takes over.

Erotica and porn can help expand your erotic repertoire by turning you on to things you weren't aware of previously. They can teach you new positions, equip you with new scenarios to fantasize about, and give you fuel for a conversation with your lover about turn-ons and turnoffs. Watching porn can put you in the mood to masturbate or just make you feel sexier in general.

Erotica and porn are handy tools that you can choose to use or not. There's nothing wrong with enjoying them, so don't be shy. The trick is to figure out what you like; there's so much out there to choose from that it can be a little overwhelming.

Erotic Writing

Reading erotic literature allows you to contribute your own visuals to a sexual scenario. This means you are never subjected to images you don't like, and the characters are always your type. Written erotica is easy to find; there are large online databases of erotic stories contributed by readers. A simple search for "erotic literature" will likely turn up hundreds. The sheer volume of material is likely to be daunting, though many databases have stories organized by sex act and sexual orientation. The drawback to online erotica is that you'll end up searching through a lot of dreck before you find something you like. If good writing is important to you, you'll have better luck heading to the bookstore, either online or in your city. Erotica anthologies aimed at women are very popular, and there are a wide variety to choose from. Do a preliminary search on Amazon, or simply head to your local bookstore and ask someone to point you to the erotica section.

One great way to enjoy reading erotica is to work it into a self-care date. Carve out some private time, a whole evening if you can. Make yourself a healthy dinner, pour some wine, and climb into the bath with a dirty book. When you start to feel steamy, why not indulge in some masturbatory self-care? A waterproof vibe is great for bathtime masturbation; even better is a detachable showerhead!

SOME CLASSICS OF EROTIC LITERATURE

The Perfumed Garden of Sensual Desire, by Muhammad ibn Muhammad al-Nafzawi

The Romance of Lust, by Anonymous

Story of the Eye, by Georges Bataille

The Decameron of Giovanni Boccaccio, by Giovanni Boccaccio

The Complete Memoirs of Jacques Casanova de Seingalt, by Giacomo Casanova

Memoirs of Fanny Hill, by John Cleland

> > >

> > >   *Madame Bovary,* by Gustave Flaubert

Lady Chatterley's Lover, by D. H. Lawrence

Ada, or Ardor, by Vladimir Nabokov

Delta of Venus, by Anaïs Nin

The Satyricon of Petronius Arbiter, by Petronius

Memoirs of a Beatnik, by Diane di Prima

The Story of O, by Pauline Réage

Venus in Furs, by Leopold von Sacher-Masoch

Kama Sutra: The Erotic Art of Love and Sex, by Mallanaga Vatsyayana

Watching Porn

More women than ever are watching porn. Every time I open a magazine, I see an article about it. Clearly, we watch porn, make porn, star in porn, collect porn, trade porn, you name it. In fact, I googled "women watching pornography" while writing this chapter, and the first two things that came up were O, *The Oprah Magazine* and CNN—can't get much more mainstream than that.

Porn, specifically porn videos, gets heavily criticized as a form, especially by those not particularly familiar with it. Sure, criticisms that pornos lack in plot, character development, dialogue, production value, etc., are valid, but we can apply those same criticisms to popular television shows and blockbuster films.

Certainly, there is plenty of bad, demeaning, sexist, misogynistic porn, but there is also plenty of bad, demeaning, sexist, misogynistic TV. It doesn't mean the whole genre is bad, though—just that you need to seek out the good stuff.

CHOOSING PORN

J. D. Ackerman is a new media sex educator and sexuality writer with a Masters of Education in Human Sexuality. She works online creating a sex-positive community with HotMoviesForHer.com, a video-on-demand adult movie site specifically for women. Use the lists of suggestions and video reviews on this site to watch either alone or with a partner.

DIRTY-MOVIE NIGHT

Why not have a dinner-and-a-movie night with your lover, only instead of watching *The Bourne Identity* for the third time, you guys can snuggle on the couch with a little smut? Plan it like any other date night: Order in, wear something slinky, and keep an open mind. It's best to pick the movie in advance so there's no laughing at each other's choices while scrolling through a list of adult films on demand.

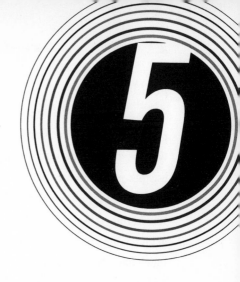

YOUR BODY

I N ORDER TO be really comfortable with your sexuality, it helps to understand your body. Our bodies are so well designed, and yet our genitals are hidden in such a way that our lovers probably have a better idea of what we look like than we do ourselves. It's no surprise that many women know nothing about the inner workings of their sex organs; inspecting them requires props, like a hand mirror and good light. You need space and time alone to learn about yourself. And even with time and the right tools, much of our sexual anatomy is hidden away, tucked up inside and out of view.

The more you know about your body, the more you can appreciate it. And when you appreciate it, your pride will rub off on your lover. If you learn to love your body, you'll be more comfortable in bed, more sexually responsive, and more connected to those responses. In fact, a 2009 study out of Indiana University and published in the *International Journal of Sexual Health* showed that women who had a positive image of their genitals were likely to have more satisfying sexual experiences, have easier and more orgasms, and take better care of their sexual health.

So let's take a tour, shall we?

DESIGN

What a well-designed organ your vagina is. It's a multitasker, a place of pleasure, a responsive, sensitive site full of potential. It's where babies come into the world and where menstrual blood escapes every month. It can expand around a baby's head, a cock, a dildo, or a fist and still clench around a finger. It's a self-lubricating, self-cleaning organ with its own ecosystem. Naturally acidic, your vag has a pH similar to that of wine or yogurt. And much like yogurt, it's full of lactobacilli, which keep us healthy by fighting off harmful bacteria. A healthy pussy tastes slightly tart and smells sweet and a little piquant.

Jokes about bad-smelling vaginas are so fourth grade, though that doesn't make us immune to them. An off smell means something is wrong. Some invader has possibly taken hold and upset the works. If your smell changes to something unpleasant and unfamiliar, your body is telling you that a trip to the gyno is in order.

WHAT TO CALL IT

Most of us mistakenly use the word "vagina" when we actually mean "vulva." Technically, your vagina is actually just the internal canal, and your genitals are more than just a hole. When you're referring to everything—and that includes the mons, clitoral hood, clitoral glans, labia majora, labia minora, and vaginal entrance—the proper term is "vulva."

While it's good to know the proper terms for everything, you'll probably feel more comfortable with a word of your own choosing. Personally, I like the word "pussy." "Cunt" is a great word, too, but I prefer "pussy" in intimate moments. It's a little bit naughty without being completely indelicate. There are lots of cute names, too—"hoohoo," "vajayjay," etc.—and if cute turns you on, go for it. If I'm sitting around with a group of friends discussing sex, I'm more apt to use a raunchier term, like "snatch" or "chach," but that's simply for effect. For now, since we're all grown-ups here, I'm going to go with "pussy," but you should feel free to choose your very own.

MAKE AND MODEL

We've all got pretty much the same basic parts, but the design of each model is totally different. If you are friendly with your body, you may have a good idea about what's going on, but every pussy is different. If you sleep with women, you already know this, and if you sleep with men, it's something you should make them aware of. Your lover can't please you if he or she doesn't know which parts deserve the most attention.

And you can add to that the fact that many of us have a complicated relationship with our genitals. Some women with a more masculine gender presentation don't feel comfortable with their pussy because it reminds them of a femininity that they feel doesn't fit them. Some women experience shame about their genitals' appearance, wishing their labia were shorter or their clitoris were less protruding. Some women are born without vaginas at all. And, dishearteningly, one out of every four girls is sexually abused before the age of eighteen. Survivors of childhood sexual trauma often struggle to have a positive experience with their body. With all these factors, it's not surprising that we don't fully understand the workings of our genitals and how to find the most pleasure in them.

Your Vulva

The visible parts of your pussy begin at the *mons pubis*. It's also known as the mons veneris, the mound, the mount, and the mound of Venus. It's the delightful triangular area right in front. The mons is covered by hair, unless you decide to remove it. It's fleshy and cushioned by fatty tissue beneath the skin that protects the pubic bone. It's a very sexually sensitive spot, full of nerve endings. Light stroking and petting of this area can feel lovely. Tapping it, spanking it, rubbing it, and the like will send all sorts of delicious shock waves to your clit.

Next we have the outer labia, or *labia majora*. The skin here is very soft, and the lips can be fleshy and mostly closed, or flat and slightly parted, exposing more of the inner lips and clitoral hood. The labia majora are also covered in hair, unless you remove it. Some women shave or wax them because they find that doing so increases their sensitivity.

The inner lips, or *labia minora,* are delicate folds of hairless tissue and come in any shade from pink to brown. They are extremely sensitive and usually asymmetrical. Some women's labia minora are long and extend past the outer lips, and others are very small and remain tucked away. The inner labia fill with blood when a woman is aroused, and will swell and darken. Between our labia minora, at the very apex where they meet, is our *clitoris,* or clit. This is the most sensitive spot of our genitals and has four times as many nerve endings as a penis. That's about eight thousand nerve endings—more than any structure in the human body. Clits come in a range of sizes, from very tiny and not easy to find to nearly as large as your thumb.

Cliterally Speaking

The visible part of our clit is the *glans*. It's usually draped in folds of tissue called the *hood*. Beneath the hood and above the glans is the *shaft*. (For clarity, throughout this book, when I discuss the clit, I am referring to the glans, or visible nub.)

While only a small amount of the clitoris is visible, it's actually a large, complex organ. It's hard to believe, but from about the 1800s through 1981, doctors described the clitoris as simply the visible bump and no surrounding parts, and seemed to have no understanding of the network of tissue that makes up the rest of the clit.

Interestingly, from the 1600s to the 1800s, the clitoris was seen as similar to the penis, only inverted. And *technically*, the experts were right about that. The clitoris and the penis are roughly the same in size, made up of the same tissue, and all parts of one are analogous to the other. The labia majora, as mentioned above, are composed of the same tissue that makes up the scrotum.

A fetus starts out with undifferentiated tissue that appears female by default. The genitals don't differentiate until after the eighth week, when the fetus is exposed to estrogenic or androgenic hormones. Exposure to androgens, or what we think of as male hormones, sends signals that cause the tissue to grow larger externally, creating a penis.

If the fetus is exposed to a mix of hormones, or if certain processes occur or don't during development, the fetus will develop genitals that fall along a spectrum of both male and female or neither male nor female, depending on how you look at it.

Because our genitals all start out as female and remain that way unless they are exposed to androgenic hormones, exposing them to testosterone later in life will still stimulate their growth. Trans men, or female-to-male trans men, who take testosterone can develop huge clits that look essentially like slightly smaller-than-average penises. For the record, an average male penis is five inches long; trans men's clits often grow to somewhere between three and four inches.

In 1966, Masters and Johnson described the clitoris as a much more extensive organ, though the significance of their explanation didn't really catch on. According to *The Clitoral Truth,* by Rebecca Chalker, it took a feminist psychiatrist to explain what Masters and Johnson had alluded to. And then finally, in 1981, the Federation of Feminist Women's Health Centers detailed the precise anatomy of the clitoris, eventually documenting the information in the groundbreaking book *A New View of a Woman's Body.*

Now we understand that the clitoris extends throughout the entire genital region. If you were to look beneath the skin of the vaginal walls, you would see the way in which parts of the clitoris surround the vaginal canal, accounting for the pleasure and occasional orgasms women experience during penetration. (However, keep in mind that while orgasm from penetration is certainly possible, the majority of women require direct stimulation to the head of the clitoris to come.)

The shaft of the clitoris extends up toward the mons and then forks and bends around, forming two wishbone-shaped legs, or the clitoral *crura*. The crura run down either side of the vagina about three inches, just behind the labia.

Starting from the point where the shaft and crura meet, there are another two extensions—the *clitoral bulbs*. The clitoral bulbs extend down underneath each of the labia minora. They are bigger than the crura and fill with blood during arousal.

Below the clit you'll find the *urethral opening*. This is where urine leaves the body. It's also where you ejaculate from if you are the squirting type. In both women and men, the urethra is surrounded by a ring of spongy tissue that fills with fluid during arousal. The spongy tissue is called the urethral sponge or the *G-spot*, which we'll discuss more in depth in just a minute. Below the urethra is the *vaginal entrance*. We think of the vagina as a tube, but really, the walls of your vagina lay flat against each other until you are aroused.

The Vagina

The walls of your vagina are mucus membranes. They remain moist even when you aren't aroused. The vaginal discharge that feminine-hygiene commercials would have us so worried about serves a purpose, but this whitish or clear substance is nothing dirty, awful, or embarrassing. This slow trickle is what keeps the vagina clean. It flushes out the works. Which, of course, means you don't need to do that sort of thing manually. Douching is unnecessary. Douching is silly. Douching is mostly out of fashion, and yet every time I'm browsing the feminine-hygiene aisle for tampons, there it is—the douche section. There are douches, sprays, scented wipes, special cleansing products to add to your bath, and all sorts of other products to deodorize and sanitize a lovely, clean, nice-smelling body part. Don't buy them. These products do the exact opposite of what they advertise. All that gunk with its perfumes and additives and promises of smelling like summer rain will upset your natural balance, killing off the good lactobacilli and leaving you open to infection.

Size

Vaginas vary greatly in size and shape, but there's really no such thing as a big vagina. It just doesn't work that way. The myth of the loose pussy is something that's propagated by our phallus-obsessed culture. It's a backward, misogynistic joke designed to distract us from society's biggest fear: that the male organ may not be the be-all and end-all of women's sexual pleasure. Intercourse is amazing. It feels wonderful, and the average male organ is perfectly adequate. Size issues are men's—let them keep them.

One factor that does have something to do with size is a process called tenting. When you're turned on and ready to go, the outer, nerve-rich section of the vagina tightens up and gets tense, but the back two-thirds of the sexual hallway—the less sensitive section—expand dramatically in length and width. The uterus pulls up and back, and the anterior section of your vagina balloons out. Without this process, the average vag would actually be a little too short to accommodate much, but the tenting process rearranges things and makes room. If you feel like your partner is banging up against your cervix during sex, spend more time on foreplay. Once you're really aroused, there's a lot more room in your pussy than you'd imagine.

Your *cervix* is the opening to the uterus. It has a teeny opening that lets sperm in and menstrual blood out. The cervix is what your gyno scrapes when you get a Pap smear—something I shouldn't have to tell you to do regularly. If you stick your fingers up into your vagina, you'll feel it; it's like a knob. It has no nerve endings on the surface, but it is sensitive to pressure. Repeated bumping up against the cervix with a toy, fingers, dick, or whatever else you have lying around can take some women over the edge into a really intense orgasm.

The *perineum* is the area of skin between the vaginal entrance and the anus. It's rich with nerve endings and very sensitive.

WHAT ABOUT THE G-SPOT?

The G-spot is very real, although debates about its existence are largely uninformed. The question isn't whether or not the G-spot exists; the question is whether or not stroking it turns you on.

The first person to write about the G-spot, in the 1940s, was a gynecologist named Ernst Gräfenberg. He didn't name it, though—that happened in 1981, when sexologists Beverly Whipple and John Perry wrote a book called *The G Spot* and detailed good ol' Doc Gräfenberg's research. Gräfenberg was writing about the role of the urethra in orgasm—the urethra runs parallel to the vaginal canal, and the G-spot is the area where the urethra is closest to the surface, so technically the G-spot is sort of an indirect way to stimulate the urethra. I should note here that outside of the G-spot, lots of people enjoy stimulation to their urethras. Dr. Alfred Kinsey himself was into plying his urethra with all sorts of instruments, including a toothbrush, bristle end first!

It seems crazy that we can still be making discoveries about our genitals and sexual response. We've had the same bodies for what, millions of years? You'd think someone would have fig-ured it all out by now. But no, that's not the way it works. Male anatomy and sexual response are interesting to male doctors in a navel-gazing kind of way. And historically speaking, most doc-tors have been male. Also, to be fair, dicks are right there in front of your face, and it's pretty obvious when they want attention. Our pussies are generally less accessible. Female sexuality and sexual response have typically been treated as secondary to men's pleasure when not outright denied and are still, right now, pretty unexplored. So there you go—that seems like a perfect reason to take matters into your own hands.

FINDING THE G

Your G-spot is just inside your vagina, on the front or top wall. It's not very far in. The easiest way to reach it is with two fin-gers, curled and pressed toward the top of your vaginal wall. Discovering it on your own is easier with a dildo or sex toy of some kind. If you have a partner, have him or her put two fingers in your pussy and stroke back and forth along the top wall of your vag. Your partner should find a ridged area that feels notice-ably different from the smooth area around it. It may be raised and swollen, depending on how aroused you are. How does the stroking feel? Pay attention to the sensations; if you feel like you have to pee, you're onto something.

Your G-spot is not a magic button that's going to give you the best sex you've ever had, nor is it a mythical place, like Atlantis, that no one has ever found. It's just a ring of spongy tissue sur-rounding your urethra that fills with fluid when you are aroused.

It's a sensitive area, but it isn't right on the surface like the clit is. When we're stimulating it, we're doing so through the vaginal wall. For this reason, the G-spot responds best to pressure and rhythmic stroking.

G-spot orgasms can feel amazing to some people and like nothing out of the ordinary to others. In our eagerness to improve our sex lives, we've gone and created a sexual mythology around the G-spot. The G-spot is great; I like mine a lot, though it took me a while to learn about it. I can definitely say that the orgasms I have that include G-spot stimulation are different. I think the description that fits them best is "full-bodied": It feels like my orgasm spreads throughout my pelvic region. My G-spot doesn't make my orgasms better or worse, just different. It's just another part of my sexual response I've come to appreciate.

EJACULATING

Female ejaculation is real. It's normal. Not everyone does it, and those who do don't do it every time. On the plus side, it makes for a very showy orgasm. On the minus side, it makes for a much bigger wet spot and more frequent sheet laundering.

Female ejaculation is not necessary to reproduction like men's ejaculation is, though up until the eighteenth century or so, that was the general belief. The Greeks, for one, believed that conception was triggered by the mutual orgasm and commingling of fluids of a male and female partner. This was actually the prevailing notion up through the Renaissance. A popular sex and pregnancy manual called *Aristotle's Masterpiece,* published in 1680 and having nothing to do with the real Aristotle, claimed not only that female sexual pleasure was necessary for conception but that conception that happened without female orgasm would produce monsters! Blame the microscope for the disappearance of female pleasure, orgasm, and ejaculation from medical literature. Once scientists discovered sperm and its role in conception, that was it. Semen was where it was at for, oh, the next three hundred years or so.

Ejaculate comes out of the urethra, usually at orgasm, though it can happen before orgasm if there has been a great deal of stimulation to the G-spot. It's not pee, and has in fact been studied and shown to be chemically distinct from urine. During arousal, the G-spot fills with fluid. Direct G-spot stimulation can trigger you to bear down and expel this fluid during orgasm, and there you go—female ejaculation. Sometimes it's a little trickle, sometimes it's a jet spray.

Ejaculation is more likely if you bear down with your pelvic muscles during orgasm. One reason we don't all ejaculate is that some of us clench up when we come. The clenching closes off our urethras so any fluid that may have accumulated can't escape. Next time you are about to have an orgasm, pay attention to your muscles. Are you a clencher? If so, switch to pushing out instead of pulling in. It might just do the trick.

If you'd like to learn more about female ejaculation, I suggest reading some books dedicated to the topic or watching videos specifically about female ejaculation. I learned how to ejaculate by watching a video aptly titled *How to Female Ejaculate,* which I rented with my husband at the time. I don't remember what we were expecting, but after watching the video, he went down on me while simultaneously stimulating my G-spot with a dildo. Let's just say it worked. He's lucky he didn't drown.

FOR MORE INFORMATION ABOUT FEMALE EJACULATION CHECK OUT THESE BOOKS AND VIDEOS

Violet Blue, *The Smart Girl's Guide to the G-Spot*

Carol Queen, *G Marks the Spot* (video)

Deborah Sundahl, *Female Ejaculation and the G Spot*

Tristan Taormino, *The Secrets of Great G-Spot Orgasms and Female Ejaculation*

MALE ANATOMY

Penises might seem pretty easy to understand, but the more you know about sex, the better it gets. This means that knowing a bit more about male anatomy can make sex more pleasurable for both of you.

The shaft of the penis is made up of spongy erectile tissue and blood vessels. It becomes erect when it fills with blood, which usually happens once a guy gets turned on. There are no bones or muscles in the penis, so that whole "boner" nickname is kind of a misnomer.

Inside his dick are three columns of erectile tissue. Two of these columns run along the top and are called the *corpus cavernosa*. One runs along the bottom of and surrounds the urethra. This one is called the *corpus spongeosum* and is connected to the head of the penis, which is called the *glans*.

The base of the penis extends all the way back into the body. In other words, some of the shaft is actually internal. The internal portion of the penis is called the *root,* or the bulb. This part of the penis ends behind the balls and can be felt by pressing the perineum, the area between the testicles and anus. One of the reasons anal penetration is pleasurable for men is that it stimulates the root of the penis through the rectal wall. Maybe you've heard of penis-lengthening surgery? It's mainly fodder for the back of weekly newspapers or ads on sketchy websites. It involves cutting two ligaments that support some of the penis shaft internally. Releasing these ligaments allows more of the shaft to protrude from the body. It doesn't actually lengthen the penis, though; it just makes more of it visible, but without the supportive ligaments to hold it up, the penis just kind of hangs there, even when erect. No one wants this, trust me.

The head of the penis, the glans, has the highest concentration of nerve endings of anywhere else on a guy's dick, though considerably less than a clit (sorry, boys!). The glans contains the urethral opening and is analogous to the head of the clit. Though it's the most nerve-rich zone, men sometimes complain that the head is desensitized after circumcision, possibly because circumcision leaves the glans exposed to constant contact and the poor thing becomes overloaded and desensitized as a defense mechanism.

The ridge around the head is referred to as the *coronal ridge,* or the crown. The underside of the ridge, where the head connects to the shaft, is called the *frenulum* and is very sensitive. Along the bottom of the dick, running from the coronal ridge, down the shaft, and over the middle of the testicles to the anus, is a raised section called the *raphe*. Many men find the raphe is also an extra-sensitive area of the shaft.

The *foreskin* is the baggy layer of skin that covers the head on uncircumcised cocks. An estimated two-thirds of American men are circumcised at birth, meaning they have no foreskin, though, thankfully, the trend is moving away from the automatic snip-snip. The head of an uncircumcised cock is nicely protected, and there-fore extra-sensitive. Keep this in mind and use it to your advantage!

The testicles hang behind the dick in a fleshy sac called the scrotum. Testicles vary in size and are temperature sensitive; they need to be a few degrees cooler than body temperature in order to do their job, which is to produce sperm. In order to keep cool, the balls move up and down in the scrotum in a sort of self-regulating AC system. And, yes, this is the reason for shrinkage. When a guy gets out of a freezing pool, his balls pull up against his nice, warm body for safety.

Balls are very sensitive to pain, although a lot of guys get into CBT, or cock and ball torture. You can buy all sorts of fun things for balls, including ball stretchers, cock cages, and weights and clamps to attach to your scrotum.

The *vas deferens* are two small tubes that connect the *epididymis* (a sort of storage facility for sperm) to the urethra. The vas deferens are what get cut during a vasectomy. The *seminal vesicles* sort of sound like something from catechism school, but really, they are just glands that produce nutrients for semen.

Semen, or cum (or maybe come, depending on what diction-ary you are using), is the fluid that squirts out when men ejacu-late. The testicles make the sperm, and when a man is turned on the sperm move out of the testes into the epididymis, then through the vas deferens and then into the urethra, where they mix it up with a couple of bodily fluids to produce semen. This mixture is expelled through a man's urethra when he ejaculates.

The *prostate gland* produces some of the fluid that helps transport sperm. It's located behind the pubic bone, below the bladder, and is analogous to the female G-spot.

HARD-ONS

The muscles that control the blood supply to the penis are normally tense and keep the blood flow at bay, until a guy gets excited, at which point they relax and allow blood to flow into his dick. As the dick fills with blood, the surrounding membrane becomes taught, like an inflated balloon. This squeezes the veins that would normally allow the blood to flow back out of the penis, creating, you guessed it, a hard-on.

An erect dick can hold eight times as much blood as a flaccid one. But cocks do not expand in any kind of direct correlation to their nonerect size. In other words, he can be a shower, not a grower, but pretty much once it gets hard, it's about the same size as everyone else's. The average size of a flaccid penis is 3.5 inches; an erect penis averages 5.1–5.8 inches.

INTERSEXED BODIES

Anatomy doesn't define your identity, and, like gender, anatomical sex exists on a continuum. There are a wide variety of intersex conditions in which a person may have an anatomical, hormonal, and genetic makeup that isn't easily categorized as male or female.

According to the Intersex Society of North America (ISNA), one in one hundred babies are born with bodies that differ from standard male or female. One in one thousand babies are subjected to surgery to "normalize" genital appearance, and one in 1,500 to 2,000 babies are born with genitalia so atypical in appearance that a sex-differentiation specialist must be consulted.

How do doctors decide what's normal for genitalia? Well, it often comes down to dick size—doesn't everything! Female infants born with a clitoris larger than three-eighths of an inch are considered candidates for surgical reduction. And yes, as you'd imagine, this often results in the surgically altered genitalia having reduced sensitivity. This also often results in a child's being assigned a sex that he or she doesn't really feel himself or herself to be.

Boys born with penises less than one inch long risk being assigned as female at birth and subjected to hormonal and surgical sex reassignment. Sounds barbaric, doesn't it? But this is happening today in perfectly modern hospitals everywhere.

The idea behind genital normalizing surgery is that children must have a fixed gender identity and anatomy to match. But who's to say what a child's gender is?

TRANS BODIES

The terms are used for trans men and trans women who have undergone hormonal and/or surgical transitions of some type but it can also apply to anyone who considers his or her experience of gender to be different from accepted norms. The term is used for Trans men (female-to-male trans men) and Trans women (male-to-female trans women), but it can also apply to anyone who considers his or her experience of gender to be different from accepted norms.

Trans Men

Trans men may opt to take testosterone in order to gain more masculine secondary sex characteristics, such as facial hair, body hair, redistribution of body fat, and a deeper voice.

Some Trans men have top surgery, which involves a mastectomy and reshaping and replacing of the nipples, in order to give their chest a more masculine appearance. Less common forms of surgical alteration for trans men involve genital reconstructive surgery. Taking testosterone (usually called T) will cause the clitoris to grow to up to three inches in length. Surgical options for genital reconstruction include vaginectomy, which is the removal of the vagina, and metoidioplasty, which frees the hormone-enhanced clit from the surrounding tissue and reshapes the tissue of the labia into a scrotal sac. Sometimes in metoidioplasty the urethra is rerouted through the head of the clitoris so that trans guys can pee out of their dicks.

Phalloplasty, which is the creation of a phallus using skin grafts from other parts of the body, is the least common form of genital reconstruction because of the prohibitive cost and difficulty. Lots of trans guys don't opt for any hormones or surgeries. These guys may bind their chests to give them a more masculine appearance, or not even that. Physiologically they may have female parts, but that doesn't make them female.

Trans Women

Trans women often take anti-androgens and estrogen, which results in a redistribution of body fat into a more typical female pattern and a lessening of secondary male sexual characteristics, like body and facial hair.

Some trans women will opt for breast implants, though many women find that the breasts they grow from taking estrogen are enough to make them happy with their body. Genital surgeries available to trans women involve vaginoplasty and labiaplasty, in which the penis and scrotum are inverted and reshaped as a working vagina and sensitive clitoris. The new vag doesn't self-lubricate, but it does have sensation and is made of erectile tissue that engorges with arousal. It is usually capable of orgasm. Trans women who don't opt for surgery may find that taking estrogen keeps them from being able to get an erection, but that doesn't mean that they aren't experiencing arousal or are not sexually responsive. Often trans women grew up at odds with their penises and never thought of them as a source of sexual arousal anyway. Many trans women learn to rewire their sexual response so that they can experience orgasm in new and different ways.

CONNECTING WITH THE BODY YOU HAVE

To enjoy sex, you need to feel good about your genitals. Easier said than done in a world where the body is so easily and frequently surgically altered. If you feel less than loving toward your genitals, maybe you need to spend some quality time getting to know them. Self-acceptance is empowering. Self-acceptance is something you can give to yourself, and by doing so you'll forever have the upper hand over your detractors. Never let anyone shame you about your body or sexuality. You can assume that anyone who would shame you about your own body has deep-seated issues of his or her own. There's no reason for you to internalize anyone else's shame. Sure, let people have their issues, so long as they do it somewhere far away from you.

LISTEN TO YOUR LOVERS

I have always loved the way my pussy works, but I hadn't thought all that much about the way it looks until I fell in love with someone who constantly told me it was beautiful. She gazed at it with such desire that I couldn't help but get caught up in her appreciation. Now when I look at it, I also appreciate it aesthetically. The mons and outer lips are curved and soft. The clit is hidden so carefully underneath the soft folds of its hood. It is a complex and unique part of my body, with so many different functions all tucked into one place.

A VAGINA MONOLOGUE

I think "vagina," is an excellent word and I confess to using it gratuitously. It's a fun word to say. As a sexually enlightened, vagina-owning feminist, I think it's your duty to say "vagina" as much as possible. Say it over dinner: "Hey, my vagina is awesome. Could you please pour me a glass of wine?"

There are people—entire institutions, in fact—that are uncomfortable with the word "vagina." Can you imagine? I know a burlesque dancer from Atlanta named Vagina Jenkins. Half the time when she's playing large venues, they won't put her name on the bill—even when she's headlining! Theaters tell her they just can't put VAGINA on their marquees. Oh, the sexism! It's so frustrating, especially when everyone seems to just love the word "penis." Now, I don't want to set up an unnecessary dichotomy, but it's just another example of the way female sexuality is controlled, repressed, and tied up in shame. These people who want to keep vaginas secret, forget it—they should fall into traffic.

A WORD ON PORN PUSSY

Pussy insecurity can affect all of us, gay or straight, but if you are comparing your genitals to the ones you see in magazines and movies, you're in trouble. Let me just set the record straight: I've worked in porn. I've worked on porn magazines and been on porn sets. I'm friends with porn stars, *Penthouse* Pets, strippers, peep-show girls, nude models, and sex workers of all kinds. I even had a few dates with a *Penthouse* Pet of the Year. So believe me when I say the pussies you see in porn have been pinkened, brightened, softened, and painted and otherwise altered with nearly every Photoshop filter you can imagine.

I once saw a magazine centerfold spread of a woman I'd slept with. Her body had been so altered in Photoshop, her pussy was practically invisible. Every part of her body looked different. Her skin had been lightened to a ghostly ivory, and her vulva looked unnaturally tiny. The color of her mons had been touched up to the point that it blended in with the rest of her body, and her newly shrunken vulva had been moved so far down between her legs, you could just barely discern the top of her outer lips.

Looking at her fake pussy in a magazine and comparing it to the real pussy I knew and loved gave me cognitive dissonance.

Image retouching aside, women who work in porn make a living off their pussies. Think of them as vagina supermodels. Supermodels have tons of plastic surgery; they get everything sucked out and plumped up. They subject themselves to constant cosmetic procedures. So do porn stars, but they don't stop at the face. They get laser hair removal. They get laser vaginoplasty or laser vaginal rejuvenation to look pink and delicate. They also get labiaplasty—a process in which the labia are trimmed to the patient's specifications. Many porn stars also get their anus bleached.

Why waste time fretting over your "imperfect" pussy when you could be out there enjoying all the amazing things it can do?

CONFIDENCE AND COMMUNICATION

Y OU DON'T NEED to have a perfect body to have great sex, but it helps to feel as if you do. Perfect, in this case, doesn't mean thin with large breasts and Barbie feet; it means a body that functions well, that responds sexually, and that does what you need it to do to enjoy sex. You don't need to fit a mainstream standard of beauty in order to feel confident; instead, you should work on finding a form of beauty that fits you as an individual.

Feeling confident about your appearance allows you to feel sexy, and feeling sexy means you are more likely to want sex. Confidence, you'll be happy to learn, is within reach for all of us. Self-esteem and positive body image are the cornerstones of sexual empowerment, and they can be learned, even if they elude you now. The sexiest quality a woman can have is feeling good in her own skin. When you enjoy your body, you enjoy sex.

For years now, whenever I've been naked with my partner, she's told me how much she loves my boobs. I spend so much time thinking, *My legs are too fat, my feet are too wide, I'm too short, my neck isn't long enough, my hair isn't long enough....* Blah, blah, I could go on and on and on. And yet it's always the same with my partner. She loves my boobs; she loves my eyes, my butt, and my wit. I waste so much time obsessing over flaws that I'm so sure must make me unlovable, but when it comes down to it, even I have to admit no one has ever noticed them but me.

YOU ARE SEXY

You are. I am. We all are. I'm not giving you some vapid pep talk; I'm telling you that a woman who is interested in her sexuality enough to seek out a book on it is sexy. I've been lucky enough to count many queens of the burlesque scene among my friends, and it always blows my mind how sexy burly-q dancers are. They can be big or small, with huge butts or no butts; be skinny or fat; or have blond hair, natural African American hair, or no hair, and every single one of them takes my breath away every time she gets onstage. I've seen curvy women spin tassels off the ends of their pendulous breasts and take on such sexual power it literally made me dizzy. I've fallen madly in love with sideshow performers who sported tattooed faces and made out with snakes, with contortionists, with the weirdest, coolest, hottest women you can imagine, none of whom looked like what passes for perfect beauty in mainstream media. The only thing any of them had in common was an ability to be exactly what they were. Sexy is what you make of it.

One of the sexiest women I know is former peep-show girl turned sex educator and author Ducky DooLittle. Recently, I opened her book, *Sex with the Lights On,* looking for inspiration, and at the beginning of chapter 11 I read this:

"I am sexy. I am flawed. I have blemishes, scars, stretch marks, body hair, and a big butt. But I am very sexy. Why? I gave up on trying to meet unrealistic standards. I decided to be as kind to myself as I am to others. I accept myself as I am and look to find healthy ways to be the best that I can be."

WHEN SELF-LOVE DOESN'T CUT IT

For some of us, body image issues are severe enough to negatively impact our lives on a daily basis. If this is you, don't be afraid to seek help. Eating disorders, body dysmorphic disorder, depression, and self-harming behaviors are very real, and truly damaging. Don't let dysfunction define your life. I understand that being racked by fear and self-loathing can make it nearly impossible to reach out for help. Our issues can be so debilitating we may not feel as if we deserve to be healthy. But help is there to be found. So many women struggle with serious issues, there are entire social networks, support groups, counselors, therapists, and services of all kinds to help you overcome anything that may be holding you back.

NOLOSE AND BIG LOVE

If you struggle with accepting your size, then make your first stop the nearest chapter of NoLose. NoLose is an organization that seeks to end the oppression of fat people. It is a life-affirming, sex-affirming, body-affirming group of wonderful folks who have let go of shame and can help you do the same. Trust me, NoLose throws the greatest, sexiest parties you've ever attended. You can find out more information online at www.nolose.org.

Once you've joined NoLose, you'll want to pick up a copy of Hanne Blank's fabulous book *Big Big Love*. Blank's guide to sex and relationships for people of size is an invaluable resource. It is full of practical advice about how to fuck when your body is bigger, but it also contains some very useful information about boundary setting and getting the kind of sex and love you want, while learning to reject attention from people who may not have your best interest at heart.

If you struggle with depression and anxiety, please get a copy of Kate Bornstein's *Hello Cruel World: 101 Alternatives to Suicide for Teens, Freaks, and Other Outlaws*. There's even an iPhone app to complement the book, so you'll always have her wise words within reach. Bornstein's book reads like an intervention, and while it's not a substitute for therapy, it can help keep you from doing anything stupid while you seek other forms of help.

I feel like I can't say it any better than that.

GROWING UP

Where are you right now? I don't mean where are you physically sitting reading this book, but where are you in your life? What stage, what phase, what part of the journey? For a lot of us, growing up is a process of undoing what we learned as children and figuring out what we think on our own. Even if our childhood gave us a good foundation and our families encouraged us to grow into open-minded adults, figuring out our sexuality can come only with experience. Let's make a list. Write down ten things you find sexy in other people. You can either think of specific people and list the qualities you find sexy in them or imagine qualities that you generally find very sexually appealing.

If I were making this list, I would say:

1. Intelligence
2. The ability to take control
3. Physical strength
4. Style
5. A hilarious sense of humor
6. Confidence
7. Sexual skill
8. Dirty mind
9. A little bit of aggression
10. Knowledge about art and culture

Phew. That might be giving away more about myself than I mean to, but you get the idea. Look at the traits I listed. Notice how none of them are "perfect breasts" or "long legs."

Now you try it:

1. _____

2. _____

3. _____

4. _____

5. _____

6. _____

7. _____

8. _____
                                                        .
9. _____

10. _____

TEST-DRIVE YOUR SEXY

When I say "test-drive," I mean masturbate. Masturbation is a natural, fun, funny part of our sexuality, and it's an important act in an overall healthy sex life. Regular orgasms keep stress in check. They keep your libido primed and promote better sexual response. Feel free to make it special. Certainly, we all enjoy a quick, furtive orgasm once in a while. But it's also nice to indulge. Take your time. Treat yourself to a bath. Use toys. Employ the showerhead, your vibrator, and maybe a dildo.

If you are masturbating, you are being sexual. And being sexual makes you sexy. When you have sex with yourself, you are creating an independent, healthy sexuality that isn't dependent on a partner. Having a sexuality that exists outside of our partners is a concept many of us struggle with—we get caught up in thinking we must be responding to another person's desire in order to be sexual. But why should we feel asexual when we aren't with a partner? We don't question our sexual orientation when we're single. We're still gay, straight, bisexual, or queer even if we don't have a girlfriend or boyfriend. By the same token, we're still sexual beings even if we don't have a lover. Masturbation and fantasy are ways to be sexual without the presence of another person.

Masturbation is like taking a vacation alone—it grants you independence. Getting to know your body and figuring out new ways to get off teach you all sorts of things about your sexual response that you can then teach to a lover. Did you know it was possible to retrain your sexual response? Well, it is.

Try something new next time you masturbate. Don't get frustrated if it doesn't feel wonderful at first. Relax and pay attention to the sensations. Let yourself enjoy what's going on without worrying about when or if you are going to come. Let new feelings wash over you, and follow them as they move throughout your body. Does it feel particularly good when you rub your clit very softly, or is firmer pressure more delicious? Note the sensations and let yourself experience them. You might just find yourself getting off in ways you didn't think were possible.

KILL A DRY SPELL

If you are in a dry spell and don't want to be, there are several tried-and-true methods for getting your sex life back on track.

Try these suggestions:

Buy new sex toys. This will get you thinking about sex and make you want to try out your new toys. Attraction is all in the head, and people who are thinking about sex draw others to them.

Masturbate frequently. All the time. Go ahead and embrace your inner chronic masturbator. Get really serious about it. Masturbate like it's your job. Do it in front of a mirror, use toys, make yourself come as many times as you can in one session. The more orgasms you have, the sexier you will feel. And when you're feeling sexy, you will draw lovers to you.

Having sex makes you feel good about yourself. I think you'll find that once you find a new lover, your self-protective walls will come down a little bit and even more people will find themselves drawn to you. That's the tricky part, right? The minute you start getting action, everyone wants you! We're all drawn to the person who's getting laid. We think of him or her as being where the sex is.

TAKE AN OCCASIONAL BREAK

Sometimes we need a reset. If you're feeling stressed out, overwhelmed, or disappointed in sex or are dealing with negative feelings in general, it's okay and actually very healthy to take some time away from sex. Here are some things to do when you are having a celibacy break:

- Spend time at the library.

- Take yoga classes.

- Shop. Throw out all the old clothes that make you feel like a big frump, and start new with clothes that make you feel sexy.

- Read more.

- Teach yourself a new skill.

- Learn something fabulous that isn't practical.

- Work on yourself.

○ Throw a dinner party. Invite the single folks you know, and make something easy and filling, like spaghetti and meatballs. You'll have a room full of adoring friends and will feel important and needed and cared for.

You can also take classes, read, start a blog, make a film, or write a memoir. Involve yourself in things that get you out in the world and put you in situations where you can meet fabulous people. Get involved with a cause you feel strongly about.

Think of the space and time you have away from sex as a period of rest before things get hectic again. Going solo for a while means you can do what you want when you want. You can come home late and not have to check in with anyone. You can do things alone. You can go to the movies you want to see, cook what you want for dinner. If you don't want to eat dinner, you don't have to. You can get off any way you like, and you don't have to ask anyone for anything. You can have casual sex. You can post an ad on Craigslist for an anonymous trick. You can flirt. You can change your mind as many times as you want, and no one will complain. You can invite friends over for sleepovers. You can have your bed to yourself. You don't have to be single to take a break from sex. Couples can also choose to abstain for a period of time. Taking a break from sex can reset your libido. You'll feel more excited by each other after a hands-off period.

TALKING ABOUT SEX WITH A LOVER

Part of being a great lover is being a good communicator. We need to be able to ask for what we want, talk with lovers about things they want, and discuss our feelings, fantasies, desires, and emotions.

Basic Rules

1. Time and place are important. Talk about sex when you both feel relaxed and happy. Don't bring up sex during a fight unless you never want to have sex again.

2. Really listen to your partner. Listening is different than just hearing all the words he or she is saying. Don't react before he or she is finished. Don't talk over him or her. Don't bully. Avoid being judgmental. Let your lover speak his or her mind.

3. Have fun. Try to enjoy talking about sex as much as you enjoy having sex.

4. Start slowly. Baby steps are good. If you have a very risqué fantasy, it might be good to start with something that won't shock your partner. Let him or her get used to new ideas before you throw out something like your desire to be nonmonogamous.

5. Compromise. Allow your partner to counter with suggestions of his or her own. Meet in the middle. Learn to stand up for what you want without being a bully. And open your mind to things you might not have thought of before.

6. Don't criticize. Ever. Avoid criticizing your partner at all costs. Feeling criticized will cause your partner to resent you. It's a sure way to ruin a sex life.

7. Make a game out of it. Sometimes my partner and I play games and bet with nights of fantasy fulfillment. Whoever wins gets a night of whatever she wants. It's a good way to try something new.

8. Follow up. If you do bring something new into the relationship, whether it's a third person or a new toy, check in afterward and discuss how it felt. Was it exciting? Talk openly about it.

9. Be specific. If you want something in particular, say so. You'll never know how your sweetie feels about a three-way until you ask him or her specifically.

10. Be glad for what you have. Take stock of your current relationship. Express to your partner how lucky you feel to have him or her and how much you appreciate the sex life the two of you have created.

LANGUAGE AND SEX

If you can't talk about sex, how can you think about it? Language is merely a system of symbols that our brains use to identify things. If you have no language around sex, you have no real way to think about it, even in your own head. So many of our sexual problems could be solved if we taught ourselves and our lovers a way to think and talk about sex that felt expansive and fun, rather than degrading or clinical. Have conversations about sex regularly. Make them a part of your daily routine. Agree on a language with your partner. You don't have to say "cock," "cunt," and "fuck" if those words turn you off. But you don't have to say "penis" and "vagina," either. Be aware of the power of the words you choose. Different people will have their own associations with different vocabulary words.

Words Are Loaded

I had always felt most comfortable with the word "cock," until one day, in a creative writing workshop, a woman slightly older than I was explained that she hated the word, generally because it made her think of giant, throbbing, angry purple erections and she didn't want to have to think about those things. My associations with that word were completely different from hers. And though it didn't matter so much in that particular setting, it could matter a lot in an intimate discussion. Since that time, I've learned to pay attention to the type of language my partners use when talking about sex. If someone refers to his or her genitals as "down there," you should take that as a clue and approach a conversation about sex with gentle language. Language is loaded, and, according to a lot of theorists, it's also biased. It's pretty difficult to talk about female sexual desire using a language that defaults to the masculine and sets the feminine as "other." But being aware of the way we use the symbols and signs of sexuality can really help us communicate more effectively. Find a sexual language that feels natural, and teach yourself to use it.

FEAR OF OFFENDING OUR LOVERS

Another obstacle to effective sexual communication is fear of offending our lovers. I myself get struck by this problem all the time. It's not uncommon to worry about hurting our lovers' egos by suggesting a change in routine. The trick is to present the new idea in a way that doesn't make it seem as if what you were already doing wasn't good enough. The easiest way around this kind of worry is to have an ongoing dialog about sex with your partner so that he or she doesn't feel blindsided when you suddenly want to try out a new type of sex.

Bringing up your desire for something new can be a little nerve-racking. It's easy to worry that your partner will think that he or she isn't doing enough to please you. Get around this by being very clear with yourself about why you want to try a particular activity and about how exciting it feels to have your lover join you.

Remember that communication is a two-way street. If you feel upset that your partner isn't listening to you, take a good look at how you react when he or she is talking. Are you giving as much as you are receiving? Are you sharing the vocal clues and affirmations that make your partner know he or she has been heard? Communication is about listening. The best communicators are people who can still listen even when they feel attacked and vulnerable. It's not always easy, I know, but you'll learn so much about what's really going on that I promise you will find it worthwhile.

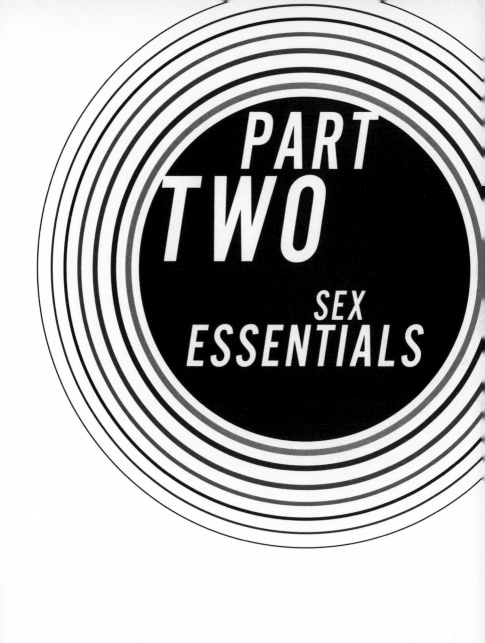

PART
TWO

SEX
ESSENTIALS

GETTING IN THE MOOD

7

THE HOTTEST, MOST explosive sex happens when both partners are fully turned on, present, and focused on each other. Foreplay is the only way to get there. Foreplay heightens arousal, increases desire, and increases the likelihood you'll reach orgasm. If you've had trouble with painful intercourse, low libido, or coming, increasing the time you spend getting turned on with foreplay may be all you need to do to resolve your issues.

Incorporating extended play sessions into your sexual activities gives your body time to prepare for intercourse and orgasm. You may not realize it, but your vagina actually goes through physiological changes during arousal: Your uterus pulls up slightly and the walls of your vagina expand in a process called tenting, making penetration much more enjoyable. Rushing through foreplay without giving your body time to become fully stimulated can lead to ho-hum, if not outright painful, intercourse. If you have a male partner, you'll find that extended foreplay helps him maintain a firm erection. So now you know. Foreplay is not only fun and arousing, but a necessary component of pleasurable sex.

Foreplay can be anything the two of you find exciting. There's no set list of moves to follow. Just be sure to avoid rote behavior. Mix it up. Do something different. Get creative about getting in the mood.

NEW-RELATIONSHIP ENERGY

With new lovers, we're apt to engage in sex play all day long; every flirtation, fantasy, and sexy text keeps us primed for sex. Of course, we don't need tons of foreplay because everything we do is foreplay. New attractions are euphoric. We focus on new lovers in an extreme way. In *Why We Love,* her fascinating book on the chemistry of love and attraction, anthropologist Helen Fisher compares new-love feelings to obsessive-compulsive disorder. In other words, new love is just like being mentally ill. Explains a lot, doesn't it?

That extreme focus doesn't last forever, though. Don't be sad—this is not a bad thing at all! Think about it: If that level of excitement lasted, our lives would fall apart. We'd never do the laundry. All our plants would die. The pets would freak out. It's not meant to last forever, and that's perfectly okay. Enjoy it while it's there, and once it ebbs a bit, work on bringing it back when you want it through focused, arousing, sexy, toe-tingling foreplay. Think about what we learned in chapter 1 about the "responsive desire" model of sexuality. For those of us who experience responsive desire more often than spontaneous desire, extended foreplay helps us build erotic tension and get to that delicious state of heightened sexual focus.

IF YOU BUILD IT, YOU WILL COME

Taking time to get turned on turns up the sexual heat in many ways, but one of the most important and often overlooked facts about foreplay is that it gives you time to build anticipation. Anticipation, and the accompanying tension it causes, is like a red-hot super-turn-on. After all, if you know exactly what's going to happen and when, there's nothing to get excited about. It's the need, the buildup, the feeling that you might not be able to wait, that really make sex hot. So don't be shy about increasing the time you spend fooling around. One of the hottest things about taking your time is that neither of you can possibly know exactly what's going to happen next.

In case I haven't made it clear, I'm telling you to get rid of your agenda. It's not about getting to a finish line or reaching a goal. It's all sex—everything you do together that feels good is sex—so slow down and let yourself enjoy it. Ditch the idea that it's all about fucking. Fucking is great, and if that's your goal, you'll get there eventually. But the more time and energy you devote to getting turned on, the more rewarding your sexual experience will be overall.

New lovers are in a constant state of anticipation. They are always thinking about the next time they'll see each other. You can create some of that new-love feeling by building each other's anticipation of all the exciting, feel-good things that are about to happen. If you've established some set sexual patterns in your sex life that aren't really serving you, like rushing through foreplay, for instance, now is a good time to start unlearning those bad habits. Wipe the slate clean so you can create new, more satisfying experiences for yourself. Bring a sense of excitement into your sex play by finding new things to pay attention to. Be creative. Explore. Go rogue.

ASK FOR IT

Be vocal about the attention you want. Your lover wants to please you but may not actually know how. Some of us are more perceptive than others, and many men and women worry that asking questions will kill the mood. Despite the well-known adage that there are no stupid questions, some questions are definitely less sexy than others. You can solve this problem by talking about your desires. If you want something specific, make it clear. If you simply need to slow things down, try taking control. Don't be afraid to pull back and stop the action or change its course. If things are moving too quickly, try something different. Direct his attention to your breasts, or tell her you want to explore her body. Touch, stroke, and kiss your lover the way you would like him or her to touch, stroke, and kiss you.

POSITIVE REINFORCEMENT

Criticism is unsexy. Use positive reinforcement to get what you want during sex play. Statements like "I love when you touch me there," "I love when you make me come with your mouth," and "I love when we go slowly; it makes me want you even more" are surefire ways to get what you need while maintaining the erotic tension between you and your partner.

SCRIPTS AND ROLES

Sexual scripts are narratives we've written for ourselves about sex. Often these scripts and roles are left over from when we were younger and had less real-life experience to draw from. Scripts are essentially preconceived notions we have about sex. They don't make sex better; they just get in the way of our getting what we really want. Do you have prewritten scripts and roles in your head? Don't worry, most of us do. Our early ideas about sex and love are shaped by unrealistic story lines in television, books, and movies. By the time we begin our adult sex life, many of us have been fantasizing about it for a decade, so it's no wonder we have some preconceived notions.

One of the most recognizable sexual scripts that affects our enjoyment of sex says that the aggressor, usually the masculine partner, is supposed to be ready to go at any time. He or she should want sex constantly, have no need for warm-up, get turned on/hard instantly, and want to skip foreplay and get right to the good part, whatever that is.

This script is so well established that when we encounter a masculine/aggressive partner who does want to take his time, we wonder what's wrong. We may even wonder about our own attractiveness, buying into the classic myth that if our partner truly wanted us, he would simply rip off our clothes, free our heaving bosom from its constraints, and ravish us like an overheated heroine on the cover of a romance novel.

It doesn't help that you never see foreplay in movies, and certainly not in porn. Sex scenes in film usually start with some movie kissing: The hero grabs the girl, wraps his giant arms around her, and maybe even picks her up off the floor and pins her to a wall.

She is ideally much smaller than him and easily overpowered, a fact he proceeds to demonstrate by dominating her physically. Additionally, he is supposed to be completely overwhelmed with desire, his ardor aroused by nothing other than her beauty and vulnerability. He needs her so badly, he just wants to rip off her clothes and . . . what? Stick it in? I guess that happens in the next scene, but, of course, we never get to see what happens next.

In the other half of the foreplay script is the person being pursued, usually the woman. She is supposed to want romance, long baths, candlelight, and slow, sensual, erotic touching. She is reluctant, maybe inexperienced, and needs to be coaxed into sex. Our poor ravishee is expected to display no desire of her own— merely a receptive, feminine passivity. She simply succumbs to her partner's desire, giving in to sex to fill his needs, because a man has needs, right?

Does this script sound familiar to you? Do you have any scripts of your own? Now's the time to tear them up. Time to change the foreplay script into a choose-your-own-adventure.

TAKE TURNS

You don't need to wait for your lover to initiate sex. If you're in the mood, go ahead and say so. Mixed messages about who should initiate are common and can turn into full-blown issues involving hurt feelings and unnecessary rejection and distancing. Don't let this happen in your sex life. Have sex when the mood strikes. Can you think of anything hotter than having your partner say, "I want you now"? Becoming more spontaneous about sex is a foolproof way to make sure your relationship stays hot.

This is just as important for single women as for coupled ones. Regardless of your sexual orientation—straight, lesbian, bi, queer, heteroflexible—if you were raised as a girl, then you probably grew up with a lot of stringent, limiting information about gender roles. I bet you, like most of us, were taught to wait for the other person to make the first move. Don't let this outmoded way of thinking curtail your enjoyment of sex. If you want something or someone, there's no reason not to pursue it.

TALK DIRTY

In our eagerness to feel sexually confident, we sometimes keep quiet when we should be talking. Don't forget, your partner can't read your mind. Fix it with a little dirty talk. Talking dirty does double duty: It's a turn-on while also being a sexy, no-pressure way to communicate sexual desires.

Your voice is a great tool of seduction. Use it to turn your partner on. Tell him what to do in whispered commands. Describe a fantasy. Whisper dirty things in between kisses. Pay him compliments. Make noise. Groan. Sigh. Get your partner thinking about sex by leaving something suggestive on his voice mail. Talking about sex before you leave for work will get you both thinking about it all day long. Say sexy things over dinner. Say them while you are undressing. Make your intentions known.

FLIRT

Whether you've been together for years or you just met, your lover enjoys being flirted with. Flirting strokes his or her ego.

Flirting makes your partner feel sexy, and when we feel sexy we crave sex. Use flirting as foreplay. Try glancing suggestively at your lover from across the table. Wait until you lock eyes, hold the glance for a second, and then look away. Casually brush against your lover while you are cooking together. Play with each other. Touch often. Try teasing your lover over the course of the evening by touching him everywhere except his genitals.

SHOW OFF

Don't be shy about your body. Let your lover see you naked. I mean fully, brazenly, standing-there, altogether naked. Your partner loves your body, or he or she wouldn't be with you. The sight of bare skin is exciting for all of us. So why hide it? Refusing to hide or cover up indicates you feel good about yourself. And that is a huge turn-on.

TAKE YOUR TIME

Sometimes in our urgency to show our lovers how much we want them, we rush through things. But sex is not just about giving and getting orgasms; it's about experiencing an intimate journey with your lover. Everything you do prior to heading for orgasm counts as foreplay. I say "heading for orgasm" because oral sex, penetration with fingers and toys, and mutual masturbation are all just as much sex as penis-in-vagina intercourse. It's important to remember that intercourse is one type of sexual culmination with your partner, but it's not your only choice.

KISSING

Nearly everyone kisses, or at least that's what we hear from anthropologists, who claim that 90 percent of human cultures kiss. Kissing is an important part of expressing affection and may also, according to a 2007 study, play a role in mate selection. Here's the deal, according to researchers: Way more of our brain is dedicated to interpreting information from our mouths, and kissing gives us all sorts of data about a partner's DNA to process. That kiss is doing double duty by both getting us turned on and decoding the compatibility of our partner's hormonal makeup with our own. With all that processing going on, you want to make every kiss the best it can be.

Kissing turns us on. It feels amazing. Our lips are densely packed with nerve endings, so we feel every bit of touch. Also, saliva contains testosterone, the hormone that triggers our libido, so kissing actually increases desire. A kiss is an unmistakable signal that things are heating up.

Kissing is also a bonding mechanism. It taps into your brain's limbic system, the area that rules feelings. When we kiss, our faces are so close to each other that we shut our eyes, transferring all of our attention to the tactile sensation. Kissing lights up the pleasure and reward centers in the brain by triggering a dopamine response. This in turn gives us feelings of euphoria and decreases stress levels. Kissing releases oxytocin, the chemical responsible for bonding and the same one released during an orgasm. And a kiss gives us all sorts of information about the sex that's bound to follow. When someone is a good kisser, we get excited thinking he or she will also be a good lover.

FIVE KISSES TO TRY

1. Playfully place small kisses across your lover's face.

2. Grasp his lower lip with your teeth and bite, but not too hard!

3. Act as if you are leaning in for a kiss, but instead hold your face a few inches away from his or hers.

4. Trace the outline of his or her lips with the tip of your tongue.

5. Suck on the tip of his or her tongue as if you were performing oral sex.

Bringing Kissing Back

If you are in a relationship where the sex has dropped off, try bringing the kissing back. Kiss your lover passionately every day. Remember how it felt when you first met. Kissing is usually the first thing to go, and even if you are still having regular sex, the amount of time you spend kissing has probably decreased. Bring back long, slow kisses. Kiss often. Kiss before bed, when you wake up, when you leave for work. Kiss in public.

What Makes a Good Kiss?

Kissing is an art and should be approached like one. Start slowly, keep your lips soft, and limit tongue action until your partner is fully engaged. Great kisses start out teasing and soft, leaving your partner yearning for more.

Let the erotic energy build between the two of you. Flirt with your partner until he or she starts moving closer. Keep the tension alive by remaining physically close until you feel as if you can't stand it and you simply must start kissing or you'll explode. If it's a first date or a first kiss or you want to make it seem as exciting as a first kiss, don't be afraid to ask. It's incredibly sexy to hear the words "May I kiss you?" Asking first can give a shy lover the encouragement he or she needs. Kiss softly until you can't take the tension; then you can give in to the urgency and kiss more deeply.

Close your eyes and think about nothing other than the feeling of your lover's lips sliding over yours. Pay close attention to the movements of his or her tongue and to the movements of your own. Make that kiss be the only thing happening on Earth.

Intersperse soft kisses with deep, hard ones. Don't be afraid to nibble and suck at your partner's lips. Use your tongue wisely. Grasp his or her top lip between your lips, and lick the underside with light strokes. A soft tongue teasing at your lover's tongue, lips, and teeth is hot. A wet, sloppy tongue with no finesse will make your lover feel like he's being kissed by his pet Labrador.

Don't stick to just the lips, either; kiss your lover's neck and throat. Place kisses on exposed skin, like shoulders and chests. Kiss the tips of her fingers. Place light, fluttery kisses on her cheeks and other parts of her face. Earlobes, nipples, and the nape of the neck are especially sensitive areas. Don't be afraid to stop between kisses and whisper dirty little ideas about what's to come. Compliment your lover on all the things you notice about him or her while you are focused on making out. Describe how wonderful she smells or how soft his lips are. Tell the person kissing you what an incredible kisser she is. Moan and make soft sounds that show your appreciation.

Use Your Breath

Breathe against your lover's ear. Lick him and blow across the place you licked. Breathe warm air against his skin. Use the sound of your breathing to communicate. Moaning and exhaling forcefully, send a message that you are getting hotter. Deep, heavy breaths will heighten your own arousal while indicating to your partner how turned on you are.

Bite

Use your teeth. Nibble on your partner's neck and shoulders. Don't nip, though—it's annoying and painful. You don't want to hurt her (unless you do, but we'll get to that later). Bite lightly. You want it to feel good, a little bit exciting, maybe even dangerous. No bruises or hickeys unless she tells you she likes that sort of thing.

Make-Out Sessions

Kissing is great foreplay, but it doesn't necessarily have to lead to anything other than more kissing. Rather than have a quickie, indulge in a long make-out session where you do nothing but kiss and whisper to each other. Kiss for as long as you have time; get yourselves worked into a frenzy, and leave it that way. Getting turned on is just as much fun as coming—you just need to change your attitude and learn to indulge in feeling aroused all day. Kissing your partner every day is the easiest way to reconnect. Spend some time experimenting to find new things that make you both crazy. Consider extended make-out sessions really enjoyable homework.

Don't stop kissing just because you've moved on to something else. Weave kisses throughout everything you do. Kiss while you are fucking; kiss while you are touching other parts of your lover's body. Kissing helps keep you and your lover present while you're having sex. Kiss his or her thighs when you are performing oral sex. Kiss your partner after he or she goes down on you; taste yourself on his or her lips. Kissing can be a great way to slow everything down and, during intercourse, to keep your partner from reaching orgasm before you. You'll also heighten your feeling of connection, intensifying the entire experience.

Mimic Her Movements

Pay attention to the way your partner kisses you, and mimic some of the things he or she does. We tend to give lovers the type of touch we want to receive, so if someone is kissing you softly, follow along with his style and technique and give him some of the same things he's giving you. If your lover is kissing you too hard or with too much force, lightly pull back and then move back in with a softer kiss. If she's paying attention like she should be, she'll back off and follow your lead. You can teach your partner to kiss you the way you like to be kissed. If he uses too much tongue or kisses you too sloppily, try steering him to kiss more softly. Pull away from a kiss you find too forceful and come back to him with softer, more fluttery kisses. Repeat until he begins to mimic your kissing style.

Talk About It

Just as with any other sex skill, to get kissing right, you have to communicate. So go ahead and talk about what you like. You can ask for things in between kisses, or you can playfully bring up things you like during totally nonsexual times. Talk about kissing over breakfast the next morning; tell your lover the things she did that you especially liked. Giving positive reinforcement means you are sure to get more of the good stuff next time around. Compliment your lover. A confident lover is more apt to enjoy sex and want more of it. Let your lover know how you feel about him or her. Tell him all the wonderful ways he turns you on. Lift her up and focus on the positive. The happier your lover is, the happier he or she will want to make you.

Use Your Hands

Add touch to your kissing session. Caress shoulders, breasts, buttocks, and anywhere else you can reach. Touch her neck; play with his hair. Put your hands on your lover's face while you kiss him. If you want to get him really hot, place a hand lightly, very lightly, across his throat. This gesture can make your lover feel vulnerable, and many people find that feeling to be a big turn-on.

Use Your Body

While kissing, press your body against your lover's in a firm, full-contact hug. Press your breasts against his or her chest, letting your nipples graze against his belly. Push your pelvis into his, letting the electricity build between your bodies. Slide your hands over your lover's back and rest them on the space where his lower back meets his butt. Pull him close to you while grinding your pelvis against his thigh.

BREASTS

Show your partner how to touch your breasts by guiding his or her hand with your own. He can stroke them, cup them in his hand, and rub them lightly over your bra. If you enjoy stronger sensations, ask him to pinch, pull, and bite your nipples. Some women's breasts are very sensitive, others less so. Where do you fall on this spectrum? Experiment until you find things you like. There is no right or wrong way to play with your breasts—just go with what feels good.

Keep in mind that we all have nipples and it's likely that your partner's are as sensitive as yours. Try massaging his or her nipples through clothing first. Tease and stoke them until they become erect. Many people find nipple-pain sensations very arousing. Nipple clamps, clothespins, and other pinchy, clampy things are fun to experiment with. We'll talk more about sex toys in chapter 11.

CONFIDENT CARESSES

The skin is the largest organ in the body. Think of all those millions of nerve endings just waiting to be stimulated. Run your hands lightly over your lover's body. Touch him or her everywhere. If your partner is female, run your hands down her back, reveling in her curves. Rest your hand on her hips. Feel the dip of her waist. If your partner is male or masculine in his gender presentation, try running your hands across his chest. Use a flat palm to explore the broad, muscular areas of his body. Feel his arms. Touch the back of his neck.

It's important that you focus on your lover's whole body, rather than simply concentrating your energy on the obvious parts, like the breasts, ass, or genitals. Pay close attention to your partner's body language. If he or she responds with groans and sighs or leans into your touch, you've found an erogenous zone. If there are places she especially *dislikes* being touched, you'll know that, too, based on his or her response.

BEING TOUCHED

Your relationship with your body affects how you like to be touched. Women who feel less confident about their size and shape may have trouble reveling in a lover's touch. If this describes you, try guiding your partner's hands. Place your hands gently on top of his and guide them to a part of your body that brings you pleasure. For instance, I feel less sexy when someone strokes my stomach, but when a lover places his or her hands firmly on my torso at the highest point of my waist, I practically swoon. You don't have to like being touched everywhere. Making peace with our bodies is the ultimate goal, but while we're working on it, why not find pleasure with the parts of ourselves we love most?

TOUCHING MORE

Touching is how we bond. It's how we feel love. Babies who are not touched fail to thrive. Touch is vital to our physical and mental health. We show affection to our loved ones by touching them. But touching can also be confusing or loaded with expectations.

As women, we're used to protecting ourselves from unwanted touch. While it's lovely to think that any touch between two people who desire each other is erotic and exciting, the truth is that touching, even by someone we love, can have mixed messages. Our partner's touch can put us on the defensive if we interpret it to mean that he or she wants sex and we aren't in the mood. Just as easily, rejecting our partner's touch by stiffening or pulling away can leave our partners feeling rejected and afraid to touch us.

This kind of cycle can really screw up your sex life. It's not uncommon in long-term couples where the sex has dropped off, but it's also possible to have mixed-message touching screw things up with casual sex partners. It's okay. If this has happened in your sex life, acknowledge that it's an issue, but don't let it continue. It's too easy to get caught up in cycles of anger and miscommunication where neither partner is sure what's happened but it's clear that something is wrong.

One fix for this problem is to touch more, and more often. Let touch become part of the way you communicate with your lover. Touch him or her in a loving way whenever you are close. Cuddle. Hold each other. Touch more in nonsexual ways. Touch each other so much that it becomes second nature. Not all touching has to lead to sex! Touch can be a way of showing affection. If you touch often enough, you can overwrite some of the anxiety-producing messages that your touch might produce. Touching more will make touch feel exciting and pleasurable again.

BE PREPARED

The best way to prepare for sex is to set up your bedroom in a sex-friendly manner. Sex is bound to involve some fumbling, but you can at least ensure that neither of you is fumbling for lube, condoms, or vibrators. Stock your night table with essentials. Make sure your supplies are clean and within reach. Part of being a great lover is being a prepared lover.

Mood Lighting

Candles make everyone look hot. Nothing is sexier and more romantic than candlelight. But, admittedly, candles aren't always practical. I've always dreamed of being one of those witchy candle-lighting women with scarves draped over the lamps and headboard. I'm not. I've tried candles in the bedroom, and inevitably I've knocked them over and spilled wax everywhere. Once, I set my duvet on fire. But if you are the sensual sort who can do candles, go for it. I envy you.

If you are more like me and can't risk a safety hazard, invest in a dimmer switch at the hardware store or buy a small, low-wattage, incandescent bedside lamp. Something that uses a 20-watt bulb is perfect. You want enough light to see by, but not so much that your room feels like the gyno's office.

The Bed

You need a bed big enough to enjoy sex in. I can't tell you what size mattress you need, but if you feel cramped, think about upsizing. You need a firm mattress, one with some bounce to it.

Extra pillows are great for helping you get into different positions. If you are a bigger gal, then you should definitely have a stack of pillows handy to prop up your hips. This will both give you more reach and create better angles for more enjoyable penetration.

Splurge on sheets, too. Thick, soft, high-thread-count sheets are a turn-on. No one wants to get laid on scratchy, thin, uncomfortable bed linens.

Keep your space neat and tidy. It's difficult to concentrate on the fun you're having when you're faced with piles of dirty laundry. Scent your sheets with perfume or perfumed dusting powder. Create a luxurious, glamorous space that makes you feel sexy and ready for sex.

FLIRT MORE

Flirting is like a social lubricant: It makes everything run more smoothly. Flirting is how you get people to do things for you, to notice you, to like you, and, most important, to take you to bed. Flirting with people makes them feel good.

Flattery Will Get You Everywhere

Flatter the object of your attention. Compliment his appearance, her intelligence, her singing voice—whatever it is you notice about that special person. Out in public, a long, slow glance and a sweet smile will get someone's attention. Don't ogle, though—you'll look crazy.

Body Talk

Leaning in toward someone with open arms says, *I like you.*
Arms across your chest and facing away from someone says, *Stay away.* Don't be timid. Approach someone with confidence and start a conversation. Listen to him as he speaks. Ask her questions about herself. Small talk isn't really all that bad once you get the hang of it. It helps you make connections, meet people, get dates, network, and improve your social life.

In the Neighborhood

Sick of walking past that guy from the gym every day on the way home from work? Stop and say hi. He's probably just as shy as you are and will welcome the introduction. Try these openers:

"Hey, don't you work out at my gym?"

"Do you know where there's a mailbox [or post office, gas station, medical-marijuana seller]?"

"Do you think I'm cute?"

At the Bookstore

You're browsing the new-releases section, when suddenly you see a shaggy-haired professor type browsing anthologies of avant-garde poetry. Or maybe it's a muscle-bound tattooed guy reading *Lowrider*—whatever works! Try starting a conversation:

"Want me to pose on the hood of your Chevy?"

"Why do you think Alice B. Toklas was so jealous of Hemingway's relationship with Gertrude Stein?"

Just remember, everyone wants to meet someone as much as you do. If no one ever got up the nerve to make the first move, no one would ever get laid.

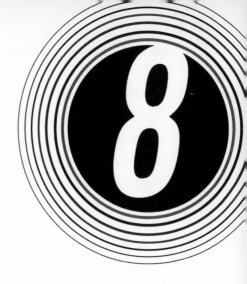

ORAL SEX

ORAL SEX IS a wonderfully intimate, deeply arousing sex act. It has always been an important aspect of sexuality, and many ancient erotic texts contain references to it. It's safe to say the act of kissing the genitals has been around for as long as kissing and genitals have existed. The *Kama Sutra,* written in 400 BCE, has an entire chapter dedicated to "oral congress."

One of the many lovely things about oral sex is that it brings you and your lover closer to each other. Quite literally, you get to put your face right up against your lover's genitals and have your lover's face against yours. It's an act of trust and bonding. Tongues are sensitive organs and tireless muscles. A tongue can feel every little bump and fold. I've always found that my tongue can find the sensitive parts of my lover much more easily than my fingers can. With a tongue, you have more access, more tools at your disposal. Using your mouth, you can nibble and suck, creating an array of sensations that fingers and toys can't match. And using your mouth means your hands are free to touch other parts of your partner's body.

CUNNILINGUS

There's nothing quite like the sensation of a wet tongue slipping over your vulva. Beyond the much lauded physical sensations, the emotional and mental sensations of an act so laced with intimacy heighten your arousal. With your lover's face so close to your pussy, you must surrender to the sensations. When you are getting your pussy licked, face it—you can't do anything other than lie there and get it licked.

Cunnilingus is wonderful, but to really enjoy it you have to let go of everything around you and just be present and receptive. Relax. Allow your partner to experience your arousal up close. Opening yourself up to that can bring you and your partner unparalleled intimacy, and what could be more exciting? Your partner gets the thrill of being right there, as close to you as she or he can get, and you get to lie back, relax, and feel taken care of, knowing that your only responsibility is to feel good. It's not selfish to accept pleasure. Your ability to do so is one of the many aspects that create a mutual bond between you and your partner.

The biggest barrier to feeling sexual pleasure is self-criticism. If you are plagued by doubts about your body, lying on your back with spread legs is apt to trigger them. There's no way to hide what you perceive as your imperfections, so rather than wasting time trying, forget them. Your lover doesn't see any of the negative things you see about your body. He or she just wants to make you feel good.

Feeling nervous about your body can ruin the mood for both of you. Wondering whether or not a partner really wants to perform cunnilingus on you keeps you from being present and feeling good in the moment. Accept and appreciate your partner's desire.

GOING DOWN IS FUN FOR BOTH OF YOU

Cunnilingus isn't a one-way street. There's no such thing as simply doing something to someone or getting something done. Any sexual experience, anything you do in bed, is going on between you. If you've ever been resistant to receiving head because it feels selfish to lie there and receive pleasure, you are doing your lover a disservice. The person going down on you is just as wrapped up in the sexy, sensory, pleasurable feeling of having his or her face between your legs as you are in having it there.

Unwind

Really enjoying cunnilingus requires being in the right headspace for it. Rather than being a simple warm-up activity, cunnilingus is really more of a main event and deserves its own set of warm-up activities. One way to get in the mood for oral sex and squelch any fears, deserved or not, about body odor and cleanliness is to start with a bath. I have always found that a presex bathing ritual improves my sexual responsiveness by about 1,000 percent. Even though I know I'm not dirty and my body needs no special ablutions to be worthy of sex, I just happen to feel sexiest when I'm really clean. Taking a quick bath or shower gives me prep time and allows me to give myself over to my lover with no reservations whatsoever.

Other ways to warm up for receiving oral sex include extended foreplay with lots of slow, sensual touching; erotic massage; reading erotica; and telling each other dirty stories. Dirty storytelling, in fact, is a great accompaniment to oral sex. While your lover is working away under your hood, you can regale him or her with a dirty fantasy in which you are both characters.

TAKE YOUR POSITION

Find a comfortable position, one in which you can truly relax. Lying down with your legs open is a classic, though sitting in a chair with your partner between your knees is a nice alternative. Keep a couple of pillows handy—it's nice to have props, and having pillows under your hips can make your pussy easier for your lover to reach. After all, you don't want anyone to get a strained neck.

Give Feedback

If your partner does something you really like, show your appreciation with groans and moans of pleasure. Let him know that he's doing a good job. He can't really stop to ask without breaking contact, so make sure to be extra vocal. Offer suggestions. If you want him to lick a little lower or higher, say so. Did you know that performing oral sex can be as nerve-racking as receiving it? We all want to be great lovers, and sometimes we worry that our sexual skills might not be up to par. So if we're doing it right, let us know!

Show Off

There's no better time to let your inner sex goddess out to play than when you are flat on your back with someone's face between your legs. Your lover wants to know you are enjoying yourself, so feel free to grind your hips against his or her mouth or to move your hips up or down to give your partner better access to your pussy. The more positive feedback you give your lover, the more eager to please you he or she will be.

Be Selfish

Forget hurrying. Forget everything except feeling good. Think about it: Have you ever known a guy to worry about anything other than his own pleasure while he's getting a BJ? Have you ever known a man to stop mid–blow job because he's worried he's taking too long? So why are we so plagued by the idea that our lovers are bored or tired, that receiving pleasure isn't as important as giving it? Get over it. Take as long as you need. If your partner wants to stop, he or she can let you know. You don't need to make that decision.

Be Direct

Having been on both sides, I can let you in on a little secret: Every woman is different, every pussy is different. Something that worked on one woman might never work again, and something that worked on Tuesday might be boring on Friday. The only way to give good head is to pay very close attention to her responses. To make it easier for the person who wants to make you feel good, give him or her some instruction. Tell her what feels good. Don't be shy. Talk about what you want—you'll get more of what you like, and your lover will spend less time wondering if he's doing a good job.

For the Giver

Let's talk first about what it means to perform cunnilingus. If you are only ever on the receptive end of this act, you may choose to share this section with your lover, or read it for your own pleasure, to gain a better understanding of the task at hand, or perhaps just to acquire useful knowledge you can tuck away. You never know how or when your sexual skills will be called upon.

The most important aspect of oral sex is being able to relax and be present. (Again, this applies to both the giver and the receiver.) But if you are on the giving end, you need more than just enthusiasm; you need to be absolutely present and focused on your partner's pussy. If you are distracted, she'll pick up on it. And if a woman feels like you don't really want to be doing what you're doing, she'll get no pleasure out of it. Keep in mind that all of us want to be truly desired. A woman who feels wanted is going to be able to give herself to you and really enjoy the pleasure you want to give her.

Tricks like tracing letters or numbers on her clit with your tongue are out. So is porn-style tongue flicking. No one likes that—it doesn't feel good, and it looks completely stupid. You should be too focused on the landscape of her vulva, on her reactions to your tongue, and on the smell and taste of her pussy to even remember the alphabet. Paying attention is what makes you a great lover. The more focused on and wrapped up in the experience you are, the more you'll be able to pick up on the subtle clues she's giving you about what you are doing right or wrong. The more she feels you respond, the more she'll enjoy it.

I'm going to let you in on a little secret: Giving great head is a sure way to earning a woman's undying gratitude, if not her heart. And it's really not that hard. Trust me, no one is really inept, and anyone who can't blow a woman's mind with his or her tongue is simply not willing to follow directions. Forget insecurity and performance anxiety—those are only going to hold you back. Eating pussy is actually one of the easiest bedroom skills to master. Look at it this way: It doesn't take any props or upper-body strength, and your arms won't get tired. All it takes is a little close attention. If you aren't already good at it, don't worry. Follow my advice, and you will be. Before you dive in with your tongue, take a good look at your partner's pussy. Don't stare in a creepy way, but a loving, appreciative gaze is a wonderful way to begin. Get the lay of the land. Note where her clit peeks out from under her hood, or if it does at all. Look at her vulva the way you would look at a map, and imagine her clitoris as the red arrow that says You are here. Commit this visual to memory, because you'll be straying off the path quite a bit and you'll always need to know how to get home.

EXPLORATORY MISSION

Every pussy is different, every woman responds differently, and, to make things even more complicated, the same woman might have different responses each time. Before you really get started, take a little tour of your partner's vulva with your tongue. One way to enhance the pleasure a woman will get out of oral sex is to make sure she's really aroused before you make contact with her clit. Tease her, make her wait—she'll only want it more. The longer you tease, the more intense that first contact is going to be.

You can tease her by spending time kissing and caressing her inner thighs and abdomen, her outer lips, her perineum, or her vaginal opening. Really, lick anywhere you can reach, but hold off on touching her clit. Let that tension build as long as you can stand it.

Start with light licks over her inner labia, using your tongue to separate them. Suck them lightly. Then move around to various areas of her vulva with your tongue, making light contact in as many different places as you can. Pay attention to her responses; when you hit something extra-sensitive, her sounds and movements will let you know. Lightly lick the base of her vaginal opening, dipping your tongue into her vagina just the slightest bit. These light touches serve two purposes: You'll get all sorts of feedback from her about which places are her most sensitive, and the constant indirect touching will leave her practically begging for it.

ORCHESTRAL MOVEMENTS

Think of her vulva as an orchestra. Okay, this just might be the most heavy-handed metaphor anyone has ever used to describe eating pussy, but just go with me here. So, are you picturing an orchestra? Good. Can you get beautiful music from just the strings section? Sure, of course. A violin solo can be incredibly beautiful. But imagine the depth and breadth of sound that come during the overture, when every instrument section is engaged at once. Your goal is to engage every part of your lover's pussy, building her up to that sensational swell and then sustaining it until she crests. When she's there, you'll know it. And that's when you bring up the first violin, meaning your tongue is sustaining a clear, focused rhythm on her clit. That's when the crest will break and she'll come crashing down, her orgasm spilling beautifully against your lips and tongue.

Keep in mind that no matter where you begin or how you get there, once she's close, every woman needs direct, rhythmic stimulation to her clit in order to come. So once you've built her up, find a beat and stick with it.

STEP BY STEP

With attention and practice, you'll figure out what works and come up with your own moves, but you should still have some basics to start with. It's perfectly okay to talk during oral sex, but once you really get going, you won't want to pull your mouth away from her clit. The time to ask questions is at the beginning, when you are building her up and turning her on. A simple "Does this feel good?" will get you pretty far. She probably wants to give you directions, so by asking her what she likes, you'll signal to her that you are open to listening.

Some women will take the lead and tell you exactly what they like and how to do it, but many of us are reticent when it comes to giving explicit directions. Even if we want to, we're afraid of hurting a lover's ego or being seen as greedy or bossy. So make it easy on her by asking. If you ask, she has to answer. It's a sexy way to get her to give you information you need and that she wants you to have. Make sure to pay attention to what she says. If she says "harder," for Christ's sake, do it harder.

Assuming you've warmed her up with light tongue contact and you've teased her long enough to leave her breathless, move on to firmer, more direct stimulation. A wide, flat tongue run firmly from the base of her vagina up and over her clitoral hood will feel delicious. Try doing this a few times in a row, literally licking her like an ice-cream cone. This will stimulate every part of her vulva at once while also relaxing her and allowing her to melt into the sensation.

If you feel any resistance on her part—if her body is tense or she isn't giving you the absolute green light to go ahead—you'll need to spend more time on slow, indirect licks until she seems more receptive and excited. Try adding some outside touching, reaching up to touch her breasts or running your hands over the curve of her hips, so she knows you are really there. One common complaint women have about receiving oral sex is that their lover's face is far away, hidden down between their legs, and the lack of eye contact and kissing can leave the receiver feeling lonely. Touching her body with your hands as you warm her up can help remind her that you are just as close to her as if you were lying beside her.

Once you've coaxed her into a state of bliss, you can stop being so tentative with your moves. Swirl your tongue up and over the hood of her clit and make circular motions around it. Your tongue should make direct contact with her clit at the bottom of your circle, and then indirect contact when you are at the top and are moving across her clitoral hood. When she really starts getting into it, try pulling her labia apart by placing your thumbs on either side of her labia majora and spreading her wide open. This will give you greater access to her clit and pull back her hood, increasing her sensitivity. You can also encourage her to spread her pussy open with her own hands. If she feels shy, let her know how much it turns you on to see her splayed open. Groan and moan and lick away with such alacrity that she won't be able to refuse.

TECHNIQUES

- o Experiment with tongue strokes. Try licking above, below, and next to her clitoris in between licking it directly.

○ Insert one or two fingers into her vagina and press against the front wall, behind her clitoris, with firm petting strokes.

○ Grasp her clitoris between your lips and suck on it gently.

○ Purse your lips and drag them all over her clit.

○ Lick all over her vulva, paying extra attention to her vaginal opening and the area just above her urethra.

STAY PRESENT

Continue to keep up steady contact with her clit. Your focus should be razor sharp; your attention to what you are doing should be practically meditative. If your mind is wandering, you shouldn't have a pussy in your mouth. If you truly have trouble focusing, try using some Tantric tricks: Visualize the energy coming from your mouth to her pussy as a circle, and then see yourself passing the energy between the two of you. As your tongue touches her clit, visualize sexual energy going into her clit and coming back out through her navel, returning into you through your forehead and exiting through your tongue. Feel this energy circle, flowing from you into her and back into you. Focus your mind on the transfer of erotic energy, and let that feeling draw you more deeply into the experience or orgasm you are about to share with her.

You should be having fun, but not too much fun. Meaning, don't get so into licking her pussy that you lose sight of the task at hand. My partner, bless her, had the most beautiful yet frustrating habit of coming while she was going down on me during the first six months of our relationship. While I admit it's absolutely the hottest thing in the world to have someone get off while she's eating your pussy, it did tend to distract her at the most inconvenient times. Unless you can time it so that you come as she's coming, politeness dictates that this is the receiver's time to come, and your orgasm can wait.

Pay attention to her responses. You'll need to switch up your tempo and direction from time to time; if you do the exact same thing for too long, it will lose its effectiveness. Just don't break contact. Switch from swirls to a side-to-side motion, then go up and down, then go back to circular licks. Pay attention to the way she's moving her hips; if she's tilting her pelvis up, she's trying to get you to move your tongue a little lower. If she's pressing her hips down into the bed she wants you to move higher. If she's really bucking against your face, you're on the right track. Keep it steady and keep going—when she's close to coming, she'll let you know. Some women will become silent before they orgasm, as every bit of their attention is focused on the sensation you are creating. Some women will breathe more heavily and quickly or will moan; some will scream and pull your hair. But regardless of what type of reaction your partner has, she will give you a sign of some kind, a change in her response that signals she's about to break.

MULTIPLES

If your partner is multiorgasmic, extended bouts of oral sex are a delightful way to make her come several times. Try maintaining contact with her clit for the duration of her orgasm. Back off a bit after she peaks, and focus more on a space above, below, or to the side of her clit. Continue to lick her lightly, without direct clitoral contact, until you feel her orgasm building again, at which point you can switch to more direct contact with her clit. Alternate between direct and indirect contact, letting her orgasms build and crest, for as long as you both can take it.

RIMMING

Analingus, or rimming, as it's commonly called, is another way to give and get pleasure from oral sex. Your asshole is rich with nerve endings, and while rimming offers more subtle pleasure than cunnilingus, the taboo factor of having a mouth on your ass can send you flying into orbit.

Rimming is not necessarily about having an orgasm. It feels wonderful to both give and receive rim jobs, but they're not meant to be a goal-oriented activity. It's more about exploration and heightening arousal, getting you and your partner turned on and ready for what comes next. If you want to have an orgasm from rimming, combine it with masturbation—touch your clit with your fingers or use a vibrator.

Before you can enjoy the pleasure of rimming, though, you have to let go of hang-ups about the ass. The biggest obstacle to enjoying anything to do with your ass is fear of its being a dirty place. Let me just put your mind at ease: A freshly washed anus is perfectly clean. It's certainly as clean as a vagina, and we just had an entire conversation about licking that.

Shower beforehand. Wash your ass well with soap and warm water, and wash an inch or so inside with a soapy finger. A tongue cannot penetrate an ass far enough to encounter anything untoward, so if you are showered and clean, you have nothing to worry about. There are all sorts of ways to clean your ass in preparation for anal play, which I'll discuss a little later, when we talk about fucking. But for rim jobs, all you need is a good hot shower. You can also use a dental dam or Saran wrap over your partner's butthole if you want extra protection.

Relax Your Butt

We are an ass-clenching culture. We all walk around with our asses clenched at all times. We store our tension in our asses. Think about your butthole right this second—are you clenching it? I bet you are. Force yourself to let go. Take a deep breath, let it out, and try to relax your asshole as you exhale. Then try clenching your asshole and releasing it several times in rapid succession.

Your tongue, lips, breath, and teeth, as well as your hands and body, can all work together to turn you into a butt-loving machine. Nibble her ass cheeks and rub her thighs, butt, torso, breasts—whatever you can reach. The asshole itself is dense with nerve endings and incredibly sensitive. Don't bite too hard, but don't treat her like a porcelain doll, either. Let her feel your desire, and she'll feel more desire herself.

For its size, the tongue is the strongest muscle in the body. Think of all the ways it can move. Though soft, steady licks will probably become the centerpiece of your technique, don't be afraid to mix it up a bit. Circles, darting licks, and sinuous tongue twists will all spice things up. If your sweetie likes featherlight touches behind her knees and on her feet, encourage her with a similarly light touch on her rosebud. Lap her up like a kitty with a saucer of milk, or ravish her like a dog with a bone.

Rimming is easily incorporated into cunnilingus. The space between the ass and the cunt, the perineum, loves to be licked, and rimming makes a good warm-up for anal penetration. If you want to fuck your lover in the ass, rimming can soften her up so that the penetration is more pleasurable. Just a note: Rimming is best done before anal fucking and not after, because no matter how well you shower, fucking can drag bacteria from inside the body to the surface.

FELLATIO

"The End. And Deep Throat to you all" is the last line of the 1972 porn flick *Deep Throat*, the first pornographic movie to become a cultural phenomenon. The movie ushered in the golden age of porn. It was the epitome of "porn chic," it made Linda Lovelace a household name, and it became the code name of Woodward and Bernstein's secret Watergate source.

Deep Throat tells the story of a woman who, suffering from a lack of orgasms, makes a visit to her doctor. Upon examining her, the inquisitive physician finds that her clitoris is buried deep in her throat. Surprise! Her frigidity issues are solved—she just needs to suck more cock. The film was financed by the Mob— New York's Colombo crime family, specifically. Made for a paltry $25,000, it went on to gross in the millions. Though the exact amount is often disputed, some claim it made as much as $600 million. We may have been giving blow jobs since the dawn of time, but it wasn't until *Deep Throat* in 1972 that Americans began to consider them a national pastime.

Men love blow jobs—no secret there. Married celebrities, married presidents, and unmarried teenagers are all big fans. Chances are, your boyfriend likes them, too. It's actually kind of thrilling how obsessed we are with blow jobs. The funny thing about their name is that they require a good deal of sucking and very little blowing. We're not exactly sure where we got the term, though it's likely we borrowed it from gay culture, or possibly from the jazz scene, in which instruments are played with the mouth. The most likely origin, though, is Victorian—back then, it was referred to as a "below-job."

PUT IT IN YOUR MOUTH

Performing oral sex, also called giving head or giving a blow job, is a great way to feel more intimate with your lover. It can give you a sense of power and make you feel in charge, lusty, naughty, and sexy. With a little confidence, giving head can be as much fun for you as it is for him. If you feel nervous and shy, don't worry—all you really need are a few clever tricks to give your man great oral sex.

Positions

Until someone invents an ergonomic oral-sex station that doubles as an attractive divan, your best bet is to spend a minute or two finding a comfortable position. I'm a big believer in sucking cock on your knees (it puts less strain on your back), though kneeling over your lover while he's reclining will give you more access to other parts of his body. It can be fun to have him sit on the edge of the bed while you kneel on a pillow between his legs. Alternately, he can stand in front of you, which gives him great access to your face and hair. Encourage him to watch as you take his cock in your mouth, to stroke your hair, and, if you want to get fancy, to grasp your hair in his fist and use it to guide your head as you blow him.

Kiss and lick his inner thighs, scrotum, and groin area before making contact with his penis. Allow his anticipation to build. Men enjoy being teased, stroked, and coaxed to maximum arousal as much as women do. Don't rush. Give him, and yourself, time to relax and enjoy it. Basic blow job moves are simple; just moving your warm, wet mouth up and down his shaft will bring him a great deal of pleasure. This doesn't mean, however, that you can't get fancy. Performing oral sex is not simply a passive act. It is actually an incredibly powerful and deeply sexual thing to do. You'll enjoy it far more if you take an active role. Take ownership of the pleasure you are bringing to your partner and to yourself.

Blow Job Basics

Begin by wetting your lips and taking the head of his penis into your mouth. You can kiss, lick, and stoke the head with your tongue to build his excitement and increase his erection. If he is not yet hard, concentrate on lightly stroking his shaft with your hands. Gently suck on the head, working your lips over and around it, until he is fully erect.

Encircle the base of his shaft with your thumb and forefinger. You will use your hand as an extension of your mouth, but also as a way of protecting yourself from his thrusts when he starts to get a little crazy.

With your hand on the base of his cock, swirl your tongue around the head. Tease his urinary opening and circle the coronal ridge with your tongue. Work your tongue up and down his shaft in long strokes. Stop and pay special attention to his frenulum, the sensitive spot on the underside of his shaft, near the head.

Maintain eye contact as much as possible. Let him watch you. Groan and make sounds of pleasure as you lick and suck him. The sounds you make will heighten his pleasure and let him know you are enjoying it as much as he is. As his excitement builds, alternate between moving your mouth up and down his shaft and circling his head and frenulum with your tongue. Follow your mouth with your circled thumb and index finger; it will feel like an extension of your throat. You can work your fingers around his shaft in a twisting motion to increase the delicious sensations.

If he likes anal play, stroking his anus and perineum with your finger can really send him over the edge. Try it and see how he reacts. If he pulls away, don't push it. But if he leans in, continue stroking him. He may even enjoy having his anus penetrated. His butthole is just as sensitive as yours; try touching it in a way you would enjoy having yours touched.

If you are blowing your partner as foreplay but still want to have intercourse, follow his lead and stop before he gets too close to orgasm. If your intention is to make him come, continue working his shaft up and down with your mouth and hand, and make intermittent eye contact.

Swallowing semen is a personal choice; most men won't care either way. It's not difficult or unpleasant, but it's also not a requirement. If it's something you feel comfortable doing, then go ahead and let him ejaculate in your mouth. As an alternative, you can use your dirty-talk skills to encourage him to come on your face or breasts.

ENJOYING ORAL SEX

Oral sex in the form of fellatio, cunnilingus, and analingus can be a an extremely gratifying sex act for folks of all genders and sexual orientations. Use this chapter as an introduction, a basic primer to get you started. Experiment with your lover until you find techniques that turn you both on. Approach oral sex like any other sex act. Keep an open mind, set boundaries, communicate about needs and desires, and be as willing to receive pleasure as you are to give it.

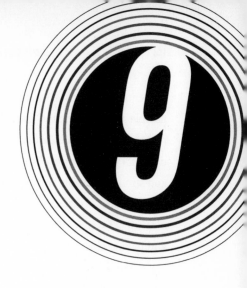

ECSTATIC TOUCH

OUCH IS A vitally important aspect of our sexuality. New research from the Kinsey Institute indicates that relationships that include frequent cuddling and caressing are longer-lasting and happier. Touch makes us feel closer to our partners. It can calm us, arouse us, and seduce us. Women with physically affectionate partners report higher levels of sexual satisfaction, while the same study suggests that cuddling and physical affection are especially important to men's overall happiness in a relationship. Funny that we've always been told that women are more interested in cuddling and men just want to get it on. These results suggest that many of our long-held beliefs about gender and sexuality don't always play out the way we expect them to.

We can incorporate more loving, sensual touch into our sex lives by learning to pleasure our partners with our hands. Our touch can be erotic or affectionate, sexual or sensual. We use our hands to show affection, to soothe, and to excite our lovers. Hands are versatile; you can penetrate your partner with one, two, three, or more fingers or even build up to penetration with your entire hand. You can use your hands to stroke your lover's erogenous zones as a warm-up for other activities or to bring a partner to orgasm at the end of intense play. Many women experience their most intense orgasms through the concentrated sensation of a finger on the clitoris. Additionally, it's easier to identify and stimulate a woman's G-spot with a finger than with anything else. We are all different, though, so the best way to learn about pleasing a lover with your hands is by asking questions, listening, and paying close attention to her responses.

There are simple hand jobs and complex hand jobs. Hands-on sex can involve penetration or not—it's all up to you. There is no right or wrong way to enjoy touching and being touched. Try exploring a partner's body with your hands as a prelude to other forms of sex. Touching him or her everywhere gives you a chance to find all of his or her most sensitive areas. Go on an exploratory mission. Find his or her hot spots, cataloging them as you go along so you can recall the information later.

NICE HANDS

Before touching your lover's body, make sure your hands are clean and well groomed. Take off your jewelry; you don't want to have to stop at an inopportune moment to remove your watch or end up fumbling around while you are covered in lube. Men should make sure their nails are clipped short and filed smooth. Nip any hangnails or dry cuticles; rough edges can hurt delicate skin. Women who want to penetrate their partner should also make sure their nails are short and smooth. Gals, unless you'll be tied spread-eagle to the bed frame for most of it, long nails and sex don't go well together.

Latex gloves are a great safer-sex accessory, and using latex gloves with manual sex makes it one of the very safest sex acts. There are other benefits to using latex gloves as well—if you intend to penetrate your partner anally, you don't have to worry about getting up to wash your hands before penetrating her vaginally. Latex gloves also make your fingers nice and smooth, which can make penetration easier and more comfortable. Make sure to have lube on hand. For manual sex, I have a strong preference for silicone lube. It doesn't dry out the way water-based types do. It's extremely slippery and leaves the skin feeling smooth and conditioned, rather than sticky. While silicone lube is safe to use with latex gloves, avoid oil-based products, which will degrade latex. If you prefer oil for body massage, switch to silicone lube before stroking your partner's genitals. It's also nice to have towels handy. Small towels or washcloths work for wiping slippery hands, and larger towels keep oil and lube off your sexy, high-thread-count sheets.

TOUCH IN NEW WAYS

Make sex feel more exciting by touching your partner in new and novel ways. Research on attraction shows that novel experiences increase our level of arousal and foster bonding. Pay special attention to a different body part: your partner's feet or legs, for instance. You can also experiment with new sensations. Use light touches if you would normally grab, or touch more firmly if you usually touch softly. Need some suggestions? Experiment with the following:

1. Take a bath together. Wash your partner's body thoroughly, paying special attention to the feel of his or her wet skin. He or she should wash you as well. Use lots of soap and work up a slippery lather. Revel in the feeling of being pampered.

2. If you aren't sure you are up for sex, try naked cuddling instead. Strip and get in bed, allowing your lover's hands to roam over your naked body. Knowing the pressure to perform is off, you may find yourself responding to this intimate touch.

3. Use your hands to stroke your partner's back, breasts, or butt during intercourse. Try lightly scratching, pinching, and slapping your partner. (You might need to ask first!)

4. Sleep naked with your partner, enjoying the feeling of his or her naked skin against yours.

5. Cover your partner's body with kisses. Start at the feet and work your way to the lips.

HAPPY-ENDING MASSAGE

A happy-ending massage, also known as erotic massage, is a serious sexual treat and fantastic intimacy-builder. When done well, erotic massage is a long, slow, torturously teasing form of sex play. A good erotic massage is all-encompassing. It relaxes people, turns them on, gets them off, and just about guarantees that your partner will follow you around like a puppy for weeks afterward. It's a whole-body arouser and a deeply sexual experience. This particular type of massage ends with orgasm, or a "full release," as they say in the business. The trick is to build the intensity of touch, stroke by stroke, until your lover simply melts in your hands. You can then bring him or her to orgasm in whichever way he or she prefers.

Create Your Space

Erotic massage requires full nudity, so make sure your room is very warm by turning on a space heater before you begin. Have the space ready. Play music; dim the lights. If you are giving this massage on the bed, have your lover lie on clean towels. You may find the bed is too low to work from, though you can always climb on and kneel next to him or her. If you have a cushy mat for your partner to lie on, then try the floor. It offers greater mobility and access to the recipient's body.

You may also want some wine, bottled water, and light snacks for afterward. Postmassage, postorgasm, postcuddling picnics are one of my favorite things in life, and I highly recommend adding them to your repertoire. Keep everything handy. It's nice to have postsex treats within easy reach so that there's no need to break the mood.

Dress Up

Why not wear something sexy? Dressing for sex is an underrated activity that can turn on both you and your lover. If you are the lucky recipient of this act, you'll be naked, of course. If you are performing the massage, go all out. Lingerie, sexy boxer shorts, lucky underwear, electrical tape . . . whatever makes you feel sexy. If I was the one receiving the massage, I'd want my partner wearing boxer shorts and electrical tape on her nipples. Actually, I want her wearing that all the time. So maybe base your outfit on that.

Give and Receive

This is a good chapter to read with your lover, so that you can both benefit from the instructions, although most of them are aimed at the person performing the massage. If you want to arrange to be the receiver of an erotic massage, your best bet is to first give one. By treating your lover to this incredibly loving experience, you are sure to reap the benefits and get treated just as amazingly in kind.

Start Slowly

Begin by embracing your partner. To foster a feeling of connection, gaze into each other's eyes and breathe deeply together. Synchronize your breathing and fall into a rhythm. Have him or her lie facedown on the bed or mat. Make sure he or she is comfortable. Adjust the cushions if you need to.

Pour some massage oil into your palm and rub your hands together to warm it. Begin with the midback, using long, firm strokes to soothe sore muscles. You don't need to be a massage therapist—any type of firm strokes are going to feel good. Pay attention to your movements; don't be sloppy or fast. Continue to rub your hands up and down your lover's back, stopping to apply extra pressure anywhere you feel tension. Think of the midback as the center of the body, and work your way outward from there. Using both hands, rub his or her shoulders and work your way down the arms. Then do the buttocks and work your way down the legs. Apply more oil as you go so that there is very little drag on the skin.

Circle and Knead

Circling and kneading are basic massage techniques. Move both hands in wide circles, pushing out from the center. You can apply pressure with your thumbs and fingertips. For broad areas, like the back, apply pressure with the heel of your hand. Mix slow, circling stokes with kneading movements. Shoulders, backs of arms, backs of legs, and buttocks all benefit from kneading. Be careful not to tickle—if your partner is twitching, you're tickling, so use more pressure.

As you massage your lover, pay special attention to his or her erogenous zones. This activity is a combination of massage and teasing. As you rub the midback, lightly graze the sides of the breasts. Talk softly. Compliment your lover's body. Talk dirty if your partner finds that exciting (and really, who doesn't?). Rub her butt and slip your hand down between her cheeks and lightly stroke her anus and vulva. Add more oil to your hand and tease his or her anus with your fingertips. Rub the backs of her thighs in a kneading motion, moving her legs farther apart. With a male partner, stroke the small of the back and buttocks. Slip your hand between his cheeks and graze his anus and perineum. Stroke the underside of the testicles. Do not speed up, and do not concentrate solely on the genitals. Make sure to incorporate the rest of the back and legs. Touch the genitals in a soft, teasing way, almost as if you were doing it by accident. This will drive your lover crazy, but in a good way.

Now Do the Front

Ask your partner to turn over. Then kneel behind him or her, cradling his or her head in your hands. Rub her neck with firm stokes as if you were lightly pulling her head away from her body. Place her head gently back on the pillow and work your way down the arms, making sure to knead gently all the way to the ends of the fingers. Then slowly work your way across the torso, gently stroking her breasts and stomach. Work across the hips. Graze the genitals. Stroke his penis a few times, or lightly drag your fingers across your female lover's mons. Continue to work your way down the body to the feet, massaging and kneading the bottom of the foot and pulling gently at each toe.

Once you are done with the feet, it's time to work your way back up the legs. Knead your partner's body slowly, staying with your massage rhythm, and push the legs apart as you rub her or him. Massage the insides of the thighs for as long as you both can stand it. Are you talking dirty? You should be. By this point you've probably built your lover up to a fever pitch. I bet she's dying for release. Way to go.

Once you've reached this point, you are ready to move on to focused attention on your partner's genitals. Wipe the oil off your hands with a towel. Bring him some cushions to lie against so that he is in a comfortable reclining position. Put a pillow under her hips to lift her butt up a bit. Make sure he or she is comfortable—legs bent, feet flat on the floor, and knees apart. You can sit or kneel between his or her legs.

The Happy-Ending Hand Job

The happy ending is truly the perfect hand job. I've adapted this version from a Tantric practice called genital massage, also known as yoni massage for women or lingam massage for men. If you don't identify with the terms "woman" or "man"—and I know many people don't—then read through both sets of directions below and combine them to create your own system of strokes to please the genitals you want to please.

In Tantra, genital massage is meant to arouse and stimulate the recipient. It is not necessarily a goal-oriented activity; orgasm isn't the point. Orgasm is, however, often a welcome side effect. You'll probably find that this type of focused genital touch can create especially intense orgasms. It can also bring up hidden emotions for both women and men. If this happens, don't be afraid. It's fine to experience intense feelings; try not to suppress them. We hold ourselves back so often, it's almost second nature to suppress our emotional response. Let the feelings wash over you, and enjoy the emotional and physical release. If your partner has an emotional reaction, stay present. Keep your hands in contact with her body and just let her experience whatever comes up. You don't need to fix anything or talk about it in the moment.

Happy Ending for Her

Begin by stroking her abdomen, breasts, legs, thighs, and arms. When she is fully relaxed, stroke her mons and inner thighs. Using your dominant hand, apply lube to her mons. I like to pour the lube directly from the bottle onto my partner's pussy, letting it trickle down her outer labia. Gently rub the lube on her outer lips. With the thumb and index finger, gently squeeze each lip, sliding the fingers up and down the entire length of the lip, lightly pinching and massaging it. Then repeat this process carefully with each inner lip of the vagina, varying the pressure and speed of touch based on what feels right.

Cover your dominant hand with lube and slide your knuckles lightly up and down the cleft between her outer lips, from top to bottom, covering her entire vulva. Your hand should be very open and relaxed, as if you were simply stroking her cleft with the back of your knuckles. Do this lightly at first, then increase the pressure if she likes it. Continue stroking her with your relaxed knuckles, hitting every part of her vulva. Drag your knuckles over her clit on the upstroke, and graze her perineum on the down-stroke. You can twist your knuckles around and add a circular motion for more stimulation, but just make sure you are constantly grazing her clitoris.

Next, squeeze the clitoris between the thumb and index finger. Feel the shaft of the clitoris, and move up and down over the shaft and hood of her clit with your thumb. Stroke the clitoral shaft several times. If she's not too sensitive, pull back her hood lightly to expose the glans. If she's very sensitive, you may need to stroke her clit over the hood instead. Lightly, very lightly, stroke the clitoris in a circular motion with the pad of your thumb. Move clockwise first, then counterclockwise. Keep up the circular motion for a few minutes, allowing her to relax into it.

Does she enjoy penetration? If so, you can now slowly insert your middle finger into her pussy. Very gently explore and massage the inside of her pussy with your finger, paying special attention to the top of her vagina. With your palm pointing upward and your finger in her pussy, bend your finger to make contact with her G-spot. If she likes this, you can continue to stroke her G-spot with one hand while caressing her clit with the other. Many women find that their clits are more sensitive on one side than the other, so pay attention to her responses and find the most sensitive section of her clit. Keep stroking her clit. Find a rhythm and stay in it. Women orgasm in response to rhythmic stimulation, so don't suddenly change what you are doing, or you will throw her off. If you need to change positions, do so and then resume exactly what you were doing. Keep breathing and maintain eye contact.

Continue to stroke her clit with the pad of your thumb while stroking her G-spot with a finger on your other hand. You can bring her to orgasm in this manner. If she becomes very aroused, she may want more or deeper penetration, so be prepared to add fingers. Encourage her to breathe deeply with you as she gets close to coming. Maintain eye contact as you feel her build up to orgasm. Back off when she comes, but don't lose contact with her clitoris. Keep going until she tells you to stop. She may experience multiple orgasms this way, or she may not. The important thing is to not take your hands away immediately. When you feel her relax, you can slowly, gently, and mindfully remove your hands.

She has just had a very intense experience, so make sure to stay present with her. You may cover her with a blanket or lie down next to her while she enjoys her afterglow.

The G-spot and Ejaculation

Genital massage is a perfect time to experiment with your female partner's G-spot and possibly make her ejaculate. Keep in mind, all women are different and not everyone enjoys G-spot play, so talk about it first and don't pressure her if she doesn't enjoy it. If she's new to G-spot play, she may find the sensations feel similar to the need to pee. This is normal; she'll get used to it and it won't feel like that anymore. You can experiment with this sort of stimulation either during the happy-ending hand job or afterward, when she has already had an orgasm,

Insert two well-lubed fingers into her vagina and curve them toward the roof, making a "come hither" gesture. Feel for the ridgy, bumpy area just about an inch or two inside, almost as if you were stroking behind her clit. When you locate the spot, press firmly. The G-spot gets firm and fills with fluid when she's very aroused. The hotter she is, the more prominent the spot will be and the more likely she'll be to squirt. Drag your fingers back and forth over her spot while stimulating her clit with your thumb or fingers. Keep stimulating it. Talk to her; check in and see how's she's feeling. Does she want more pressure? Less? Ask!

Once you've gotten a feel for where her G-spot is, continue stroking it with as much pressure as you can muster. You don't necessarily want to fuck her harder or deeper; instead, concentrate on maintaining firm contact with the ridgy area at the top of her vagina. Stroke it back and forth with the pads of your fingers. Press firmly.

Continue stroking her clit with one hand and her G-spot with the other. It's tricky, but you'll get used to it. If you find that you can't maintain a rhythm on her clit while stroking her G-spot, place her own fingers on her clit and tell her to touch herself. If she's shy, tell her it turns you on. As she gets close to orgasm, she may begin to bear down. If you feel her doing this, continue to push back until the moment of orgasm. Let her push out your fingers as she comes.

HOW TO EJACULATE

The big difference between squirters and nonsquirters is whether they push out or pull in during orgasm. In order to ejaculate, you should bear down and push out during orgasm, rather than clenching your PC muscles and pulling in. Don't be afraid of letting go. Give in to whatever happens. When you are about to come, bear down and push against your partner's fingers in your pussy. Continue to bear down through the duration of your orgasm. You may ejaculate or not. Don't worry if it doesn't happen—just keep trying. Ejaculation is more likely when you are well hydrated but not worried about urinating. Make sure to drink enough water, as well as to pee before sex to help put your mind at ease.

When Four Fingers Just Aren't Enough

Fisting is another lovely addition to genital massage. You may find that your partner becomes so aroused that she wants more fingers, and then more fingers, and next thing you know you don't have any more fingers to offer her. Lucky you. She's tenting all over the place, begging for deeper penetration—it's time to call in the big guns.

Fisting is the practice of penetrating your partner with your entire hand. It's a slow process—you don't just jam your fist into someone. You work up to it, two fingers, then three, then four. Then add the thumb. Eventually you fold your hand up, with your thumb against your palm, and push your hand past her vaginal opening. Your hand naturally curls up into a ball as you push it in, hence the term "fisting."

Fisting generally takes time and patience and slow, precise movements. It requires trust and willingness. The person being fisted has to want to be fisted. Intense penetration, whether it's anal or vaginal, is mostly about your head. If you really want something and you are very aroused, your body will be open and receptive. If you are afraid or nervous, your muscles will contract and you won't be able to take your partner's hand.

Fisting is a lot easier than you'd think. Your pussy is stretchy—and there's a lot more room in it than you realize. Your cunt balloons out and expands when you are very aroused, creating lots of space in which to fit a fist. You'll need more lube than you think you need. Apply what you think is a lot of lube, and then add more and continue adding lube as you add fingers. Assuming you've already worked up to two fingers, add more lube to your hand and add a third.

Continue to fuck her with three fingers, feeling her cunt open up. If she wants more, add a fourth. Add more lube and rotate your four fingers at the entrance to her vag to help her open up. If she's pushing against you and saying she wants more, that's a good sign. Continue to press your fingers against the opening to her vag, rotating and thrusting them in and out in a controlled way.

When she feels open and ready, tuck your thumb into your palm and fold your hand so that it is as narrow as possible. Once you've gotten this far, you are just about ready for the rest of it. Slowly, slowly, slowly push your hand into her until the widest part of your hand is at the entrance to her cunt. Rotate your hand a few times as you ease it past the tight ring of muscle at the vaginal opening. Go very slowly and add lube often. If you feel a lot of resistance, stop and pull back a bit. If you have large hands, you may not be able to fist her. If this is the case, go back to four fingers. Fisting isn't something you can force. If she's ready and really wants it, it will feel somewhat easy. Check in with her. If she wants more, continue to push your hand against the tight ring of muscle. Eventually you will feel her give and your hand will slip in past the knuckles.

Soon your entire hand will disappear into her pussy. You'll notice as you make your way in that it naturally starts to curl into a fist. Next thing you know, you'll be in to the wrist. Once you're inside, hold still. The feeling is probably overwhelming for your partner, so try to keep your movements to a minimum. If she wants you to thrust, she will let you know. Unless you guys do this all the time, she's probably pretty overwhelmed by the feeling of a whole hand in there. So take it slowly.

It's easiest to remove your fist by letting her force it out as she comes. But this might not always happen. So be prepared to ease it out when she has had enough. Don't pull out suddenly—it can be painful. Instead, work your way out of her vag as slowly as you went in. Talk to her during the entire process. You should be checking in with her about how everything feels. Let her guide you.

You can combine fisting with all sorts of other forms of stimulation, like vibrators or fingers on her clit. Or she may find being fucked like this to be so intense that she wants nothing more than to ride the wave of sensation you are giving her. Sometimes being fisted can cause your partner to ride on the edge of orgasm for a very long time because it is such an overwhelming sensation.

If this is the case, she may need a vibrator or some other type of direct clitoral stimulation to make it over the edge. Stay present and talk to her.

She may have a very big orgasm. Some women experience such a huge physical release, it also triggers an emotional release. She may sob, cry, or shake. Hold her and stay close to her as she comes down.

Happy Ending for Him

Pour a small quantity of silicone- or water-based lube into the palm of your hand and rub your palms together to warm it. Also pour a small amount of lube onto the shaft of his penis and testicles. Let it trickle from the bottle down the shaft of his penis. Begin by gently massaging the testicles, taking care to touch him gently. Massage his scrotum. Stroke the area above his penis, and caress the area over his pubic bone. Take your time. Touch him mindfully. Use long, slow strokes around his penis without touching it directly. Massage his perineum. Take your time. You are massaging an often neglected area of his body, so do it with reverence. Touch him softly, but firmly and intentionally, so that he feels your desire as much as he does his own.

Once he is aroused and used to your touch, stroke the shaft of his penis. Grip his dick with your hand and stroke up and down. Vary your speed and pressure. Gently squeeze the penis at the base with your right hand, pulling up and sliding over the head and off. Then do the same with your left hand. Take your time doing this—right, left, right, left. Continue alternating hands, starting from the base of his cock and pulling up, stroking the shaft with a lightly closed fist. Change direction by starting at the head of his dick and gently squeezing the head, then sliding your closed fist down the shaft and off. Alternate right and left hands, using the same pressure and length of stroke.

Massage the head of his dick with your palm. Move your palm around the head in a circular motion, almost as if you were polishing it. Massage all around the head and shaft. He may or may not go soft as you perform this technique. Don't worry. He'll get hard again. In fact, he may get hard, then go soft, then get hard again. Just continue the rhythmic stroking, checking in with him about speed and pressure.

If he gets close to orgasm, back off a bit, allowing him to go slightly soft before starting back up. Do this several times, letting him come close to ejaculating and then backing off. The more times you build him up and back off, the longer and more intense his eventual orgasm will be. To distract him from coming, have him breathe deeply with you.

Next, find and massage his P-spot, or prostate gland. There are two ways to do this. One is by touching the spot midway between the testicles and the anus, where you'll find a small indentation about the size of a pea, or maybe larger. Be gentle and push inward. He will feel the pressure deep inside. It is a sensitive spot and may feel uncomfortable at first. You can massage his penis with your right hand and massage his P-spot with your left hand. Try pushing in on this spot when he nears ejaculation.

The other way to access his P-spot is through the anus. Lots of guys, especially straight guys, are uncomfortable with penetration at first. Like us, they get lots of negative sexual conditioning. Penetration scares them, and they might even think it's a challenge to their masculinity. Reassure him. Then reassure him more. If he's open to it, be careful here and use plenty of lube. Make sure he is breathing with you, then slip your finger into his butthole about an inch or so. Bend your finger back in a "come hither" gesture, just as you would for a woman's G-spot. You will feel his prostate gland. Stroke it. Vary the pressure and speed of massage. He may want you to continue stroking his cock, or he may want you to concentrate on his prostate. As he gets closer to coming, increase pressure on his P-spot. When he is ready to ejaculate, encourage him to breathe deeply. He should continue to breathe deeply for the duration of his orgasm.

He will probably have a super-intense climax, especially if he's held back from coming several times. After he comes, gently remove your hands and allow him to lie there quietly. Cover him with a blanket, or hold him. Stay present and allow him to bask in his afterglow.

TOUCH WITH INTENTION

Now that you've explored the possibilities of erotic touch, you have the potential to bring yourself and your lover endless amounts of pleasure. Just remember that all touch is okay when it feels good, and if it doesn't feel good for both of you, you don't need to continue. There is always more to learn about sex, and I encourage you to explore other books and learn as much as you can about the erotic and healing power of touch.

If you'd like to learn more about Tantra, I recommend reading Barbara Carrellas's amazing book, *Urban Tantra*. Her writing is warm, approachable, full of wisdom, and at times very moving.

ENHANCING INTERCOURSE

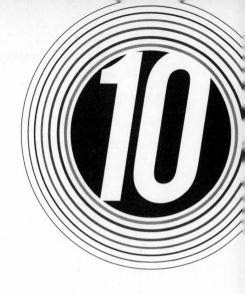

W OMEN IN THE movies have simultaneous orgasms with their partner in every sexual encounter. Women in real life do so far less often. The statistics vary, depending on who's doing the surveying, but in general, about 75 percent of women report that they do not come from intercourse alone. I imagine that the 25 percent who do are of the highly orgasmic variety, the type who have orgasms if you stare at them too long. I have several friends like this, and no, I'm not jealous. (Most of the time.)

The statistical nonanomalies among us also love intercourse, and why not? It's great fun. For me and for a lot of women— straight, lesbian, bi, and otherwise—intercourse with a penis or dildo is an essential part of an overall satisfying sexual experience and an exciting, intimate bonding activity with a lover. Intercourse is especially delicious when combined with masturbation, using either a vibrator or your fingers, and that combination often leads to orgasm. In this chapter we'll talk about positions that enhance intercourse, as well as about incorporating masturbation into intercourse as a way to make intercourse a route to orgasm.

ENHANCERS

There are a few tricks to make intercourse more fun, no matter
what position you are in:

1. Leave some clothes on. Creating some barriers to full
    nudity can force you to be creative, not to mention
    give your partner a visual thrill. Try leaving your
    panties on and having him pull them to the side
    while he enters you. The really adventurous can
    leave everything on. Have him simply push up your
    skirt and leave his pants around his ankles, kind of
    like having a quickie at the office holiday party.

2. Do it slowly. Do everything in slow motion. Have
    him thrust his penis in a slow, concentrated manner
    using long strokes interspersed with shorter ones.
    The thrusting should be so slow that you can
    actually feel every inch of his penis as he pushes it in
    and pulls it out. However, it's fine to speed up as one
    or both of you nears orgasm—this isn't supposed to
    be torture (unless you like that kind of thing).

3. Roughhousing. Roughhousing is not necessarily the
    same as rough sex; it's simply a way to inject some
    erotically charged playfulness into lovemaking. He
    can give your hair a tug while you're doing it doggie-
    style. You can pinch his nipples while you're riding
    him. A little playful pinching, biting, and smacking
    will make the experience feel new and different. The
    sharp sensation of a smack or bite, coupled with the

excitement of trying something new, can trigger the release of oxytocin and dopamine, which in turn can take your arousal to a higher level.

4. Use tools. Use pillows to prop up your hips and change the angle of penetration. Get off your back— do it bending over the bed, the couch, or a chair. Get a little kinky with props like handcuffs, feathers, massage oil, and sex toys.

5. Get out of bed. Have sex in the kitchen, on the couch, in the shower, maybe even in the car!

POSITIONS

There really is no "best" position for intercourse. Our bodies and erogenous zones are all very different—the best position is the one that gives you and your partner the most pleasure. Many of us have a tried-and-true favorite that we return to again and again, and there's nothing wrong with that. However, it can be very exciting for both of you to break out of your comfort zone and try something new.

Most positions, even the most ridiculously acrobatic, are simply versions of the basics:

1. The other person is on top, you are on the bottom.

2. You are on top, the other person is on the bottom.

3. You are on your hands and knees, the other person is behind you, a.k.a. doggie style.

4. You are both lying on your side.

5. Sitting.

6. Standing.

People have been humping each other for 4.4 million years, so if there had been any real developments, I'm sure the surgeon general would have sent out a press release, or at least written a blog post. That said, there are myriad variations on these six basics, some of which can make your orgasm a lot more likely.

TAKE CONTROL OF YOUR ORGASM

So many of us grow up with the belief that our partners will give us pleasure and orgasms, and because of this, we are often reluctant to take a more active role in creating pleasure for ourselves during intercourse. No matter how great a lover your partner is, he or she can't read your mind and can't steer every aspect of your pleasure. The receptive role in intercourse is considered the feminine role.

This is another example of the way rigid gender prescriptions corral our sexuality and sexual pleasure. Gender-based sexual etiquette favors male pleasure over female. This is why so many of us struggle to orgasm during intercourse. We're all affected by the socially constructed yet widely accepted belief that the proper way to have intercourse is to passively receive a partner's penis. None of us escapes this sort of gender-role conditioning; it's something we have to unlearn as we become adults. The reason most of don't have orgasms during intercourse has nothing to do with our physiology—it has to do with our attitudes.

Your partner should be attentive to your needs, of course. You should expect him or her to possess sexual skills and empathy, and to know how to please you, but he or she can't actually "give" you an orgasm without your participation. Sex is something you are doing together, and your orgasm is just as much your responsibility as it is your lover's. The phallus, despite what most romantic and erotic writing would have you believe, is not a magic wand that provides women with ultimate pleasure. You must take an active role. Be responsible for your orgasms. Have sex in positions that allow you access to your clit, and be vocal about what feels good and what isn't working. Change positions when you need to.

Touch yourself. I can't say it enough: Have sex in positions that allow you access to your clit, and touch yourself during intercourse. Do not worry that your partner will be offended—the world is starting to get a clue about women and orgasms. Most men understand that you need clitoral stimulation in order to get off. If he seems a little reticent or nervous that your desire to touch your clit means he isn't a good lover, give him tons of positive feedback. Make sure his ego is firmly intact and that he feels appreciated. He deserves to feel desired and cared for. He also deserves to have a partner who participates in her own pleasure.

It's likely that he'll be turned on by the way you touch yourself, and if it takes some time for him to warm to the idea, that's okay. It seems simple, but keep in mind that women's participating in their own pleasure is a revolutionary notion. On the off chance he's uncomfortable with you giving yourself a hand, be prepared to talk with him about it. Men need time to adjust to new things, especially things that challenge their role as provider. Should his reluctance persist, you have a couple of choices: You can teach him to stimulate your clit directly during intercourse, the way you would stimulate it yourself, or you can choose to find another lover.

Keep in mind that you don't need to have an orgasm *during* intercourse to enjoy it. Intercourse feels wonderful regardless, so don't stress out about your orgasm. You can choose to enjoy the feeling of penetration and have your orgasm before or after.

Good Vibes

There are many options on the market for small vibrators you can use during partner sex. Find one you like and use it. Don't be shy. Explain to your partner that your vibrator will greatly enhance the experience of intercourse and will allow you to come with much less effort. He or she will love the idea that you will be able to have an orgasm whenever you want. Vibrators take the pressure off, which allows both you and your partner to relax without fear that you won't have an orgasm. Using a vibrator during sex says you are sexually liberated and serious about enjoying sex, and there is absolutely no downside to that. We'll talk a bit more about introducing your lover to your sex toys in chapter 11.

Finish big. Many women choose to enjoy intercourse with their partner until he has an orgasm, and then finish themselves off with a vibrator while he watches. It's sex plus a show—what could be better? In this scenario, everyone's a winner.

BASIC VARIATIONS

Standard missionary position isn't the greatest for clit stimulation, though it scores big in every other category. The eye contact is great, the feel of your partner's body on top of yours is exciting, and lying there on the pillow while the person toils away is also kind of nice (admit it). Try altering standard missionary so that your lover is kneeling between your legs. You'll find that putting your legs over his shoulders allows him to penetrate you more deeply, and the angle will feel great on your G-spot. Stroke your clit in time with his thrusts.

Doggie-style allows your lover to watch his penis going in and out of you. This will be a very visually stimulating position for him. For you, it allows you access to your clitoris, and if you lean forward on your elbows, his penis can stimulate your G-spot. Try lying on your stomach so that your clit rubs against the sheet as he thrusts into you. You can also try lowering your torso and sticking your ass high in the air, which will make it easier for him to thrust very deeply.

Side-by-side works well when combined with rear entry. He enters you from behind while in a spooning position. You move your upper body away from him and throw your superior leg over his hip. You'll lose the body-to-body contact, but you'll gain a whole lot more mobility.

Coital Alignment

Coital alignment is a variation on the missionary position where you line up your pelvises so that your clit is stimulated by his pelvic bone and the base of his penis. Does it work? Well, yes—once you get the hang of it, it's great. One of the nice things about coital alignment is that it requires slow, concentrated movements and offers full-body contact, meaning the romance-and-intimacy part is practically built in. Studies show that this position is great for female orgasm in couples who have practiced and mastered the technique. It doesn't necessarily work on the first try, but if you are willing to practice, practice, practice, then there's a lot of payoff to be had.

Start with him on top of you. He should enter you from a higher-than-usual angle so that his pelvic bone is in contact with the top of your mound. You need a tight fit. The trick to this position is to maintain this contact. With him fully inside you, start a gentle rocking motion. In coital alignment, there is no thrusting; your pelvic bones should stay locked together. Wrap your legs tightly around him to help maintain the connection. Rock together and find a rhythm you can stick to. It takes a little practice, but eventually you'll build up a groove. Keep up the pressure/rocking/rhythm until you both reach orgasm.

Yab Yum

Yab Yum is a classic Tantric position. It's a variation on a sitting position and requires a bit of flexibility, though you can prop yourself up with pillows to make it easier. In this position, your chakras (the energy points along your spine) are aligned and you are face-to-face, which allows you to kiss, fondle, and caress each other. Sit cross-legged facing each other and wrap your legs around your partner's waist. You should be straddling him, essentially sitting astride him. You can put a pillow under your hips if you like. He can also extend his legs if sitting cross-legged is uncomfortable. Bigger folks or folks with reduced flexibility may especially want to modify this position by using cushions.

While you're wrapped around each other, insert his penis into your vagina. This position works very well for men who have trouble maintaining a firm erection, as it doesn't require deep penetration yet still feels wonderful for both of you. Once he is inside you, maneuver your pelvis so that the base of his penis provides as much indirect clitoral stimulation as possible. Similar to the coital alignment technique, the Yab Yum is more of a rocking than a thrusting position. With your arms around each other and your bodies pressed together, begin moving in a rocking motion.

The eye contact and body proximity this position creates keeps you completely focused on each other, which helps the intensity build. Practice breathing and let the sexual momentum increase. Pause occasionally while he is inside you to simply feel the pressure his penis is creating against your clit. Long pauses combined with focused rocking stimulation can help you both build up to a very powerful orgasm.

The Orgasm Loop

Sex journalist Susan Crain Bakos created a technique she calls the Orgasm Loop. You can read more about it in her book of the same name. She combines some elements of Tantra with breathing exercises and rhythmic squeezing of the PC muscles to build up to orgasm during intercourse. To use Bakos's technique, you begin by visualizing your arousal. Imagine it as a tangible thing, similar to your lover's erection. Focus intently on this image.

Bakos suggests picturing your vulva in its most swollen form, or using other suggestive images, like orchids and sunsets, if that's more your style.

Use this visual to help build your arousal. Concentrate on your image while building the sensation of energy in your pussy. Try to imagine your arousal as a coiled ball of energy. Imagine it as it unravels and moves into your clit. I find that this works best for me if I imagine the energy as a spinning ball of light.

Once you feel the energy rising in your genitals, begin breathing very deeply and rhythmically to help heighten your arousal. Move the energy through your body in time with your breathing. Literally breathe the energy up and through your body as if it were something physical you can move around. Keep breathing this energy in and through your body in a circular fashion. The controlled breathing and energy create heat, which you are circulating through your genitals. The breathing adds more oxygen to your bloodstream and creates more blood flow to your genitals.

Add rhythmic muscle contractions by squeezing and releasing your PC muscles in time with your breathing. Squeeze as you breathe in; release as you breathe out. Add clitoral stimulation either by touching your clit or by positioning yourself so that your clit is in contact with your partner's pelvic bone and the base of his penis. You should be very aroused at this point and require very little stimulation to reach orgasm. Keep up the breathing and visualization as long as you need to. Don't be discouraged if you lose focus—just bring yourself back to the same imagery, breathing, and intention each time. Like coital alignment, the Orgasm Loop takes practice. Don't feel discouraged if it doesn't work for you at first.

Women with Female Lovers

The three alternative intercourse methods I've described can all be modified easily to work for women with female lovers. All forms of intercourse are well suited for penetrative strap-on play, but coital alignment and Yab Yum are especially applicable to a type of nonpenetrative sex called tribading, which is the act of rubbing your puss on something—your lover's thigh or mons—or rubbing vulva to vulva, also called scissoring. ("Scissor sisters" is slang for "lesbians." Yes, the band the Scissor Sisters is in on the joke, and now you are, too.)

Ancient Romans referred to women who had sex with other women as *tribas,* from the Greek word *tribein,* meaning "to rub." The term became synonymous with lesbian sex, and *tribade* became a popular slang word for "lesbian." *Tribade* seems like a hilariously outdated term now, but it was popular for almost three centuries.

Tribading with a female lover can be a highly erotic experience. Try locking your vulvas against each other and starting a rubbing/rocking motion, as described in the above section on coital alignment. To heighten sensation, you can pull up on your mons and spread your outer labia so that your clitoris comes into direct contact with your lover's pubic bone. Bellies can get in the way, so larger bodies will need to modify this position. One trick is to straddle your lover's buttocks or thighs while she lies facedown on the bed. You can rub your way to orgasm while enjoying the visual thrill of her naked body beneath you. Add some dirty talk to heighten the experience, and make sure she stays present and excited. She can use the visualization techniques described in the Orgasm Loop section to heighten her own pleasure. By breathing and squeezing her PC muscles in time with your strokes, using visualization, and manipulating the erotic energy in her genitals, she may have an orgasm this way.

NONINSERTIVE SEX

Heterosexual couples may also enjoy a similar type of noninsertive sex. If your man has trouble maintaining an erection, noninsertive sex can take the pressure off and allow you to enjoy each other's bodies without having performance anxiety. Noninsertive sex can also work as a sex-life reset—taking the focus off penetration forces you to get creative. Sex researcher Laura Berman has even given it a nickname: She refers to nonpenetrative sex as VENIS ("very erotic noninsertive sex").

VENIS refocuses your attention on the parts of the female anatomy that are often neglected during intercourse. You can take some tips from the *tribades* and enjoy some dry-humping VENIS action, or you can make a game of it by challenging each other to come up with new ways to get off that don't involve P in V.

ANAL INTERCOURSE

When done right—meaning with trust, patience, lots of lube, and lots of warm-up—anal sex can feel amazing. Your anus is rife with tiny nerve endings, and extremely sensitive erogenous areas—for instance, the perineal sponge, a bundle of nerve and erectile tissue similar to your G-spot, is best reached through anal penetration.

Anal sex can be an especially exciting part of your sex life. It feels a little naughty, a little taboo, and maybe even a little edgy. Doing something new and exciting with your partner is a great intimacy-building experience and can dramatically increase your level of trust. Because anal sex requires so much communication, it can be a wonderful bonding experience with your partner. Many devotees of anal sex report experiencing intense orgasms more frequently through anal intercourse than through any other sexual activity. Some women who are unable to reach orgasm through vaginal intercourse have found that they can have orgasms during anal intercourse. Because anal intercourse stimulates several erogenous zones simultaneously, orgasms from anal sex are usually of the blended variety, often described as "full-body orgasms."

Warm-Up

Take your time with anal sex. It's not a quickie activity; it feels best when you are very aroused, so spend extra time warming up. Assuming you are the receiver, ask your partner to stroke your ass and thighs as a way for you to become accustomed to his or her touch. He should work from stroking your buttocks to lightly stroking your anus. He can also stroke your pussy with his fingers and perform oral sex beforehand to get you excited.

The more lube you use, the better. Position yourself for rear entry, with your torso on the bed and your ass in the air. Your partner should apply lube to your anus with his fingers. Have him tease and stroke your anus a bit, applying more lube while he does so. This will build anticipation, making the experience more pleasurable. Once you feel ready, your lover can enter your ass with his well-lubed finger. Have him go slowly; it's good to start by rubbing your sphincter in a circular motion and pressing gently until he feels you open up. With his finger inside you, he should slowly push in farther until he is in past the knuckle.

Ask him to pause if you feel any discomfort. Usually you just need a second to adjust, and then he can go right back to pushing his finger in and out. If you are going to have anal intercourse with a penis or dildo, he may want to put another finger in at this point to help your ass loosen up a bit more. Do this only if it feels good. Can you reach your clitoris? Stroke it. It's okay to have an orgasm; you can always come again. Plus, having an orgasm will help you loosen up in preparation for penetration with a penis or dildo.

Your partner should make sure that his penis or dildo is fully lubed up before he enters you. After putting copious amounts of lube on his penis and your anus, he can tease your butthole a bit with the head of his dick. Rubbing the head against your pucker will feel amazing for both of you. He can stay there as long as you both want, and there's no need to go any farther. Ask him to stroke his shaft while pressing the head of his penis against your butthole. The teasing, subtle movements, coupled with the thrill of doing something a little naughty, will feel extremely erotic. This is, in fact, a perfect position for mutual masturbation. He can stroke his shaft with his fist or, after applying more lube, slide it up and down between your cheeks. Reach down and touch your clit while he does this. You can both have powerful orgasms this way.

When you are ready for penetration, let him know. He should start by pressing the head of his dick in. Relax and allow him to penetrate you. Keep the lube handy; you may want to add more as you go. The more you use, the more fun you'll have. If you need more, you'll know before he does, so don't be shy about saying something. Anal sex can be very rewarding, but without proper preparation it can also feel uncomfortable or even painful. Using copious amounts of lube and communicating with your partner can help you avoid discomfort.

When he feels your sphincter relax a bit, he can push in farther. The rear-entry position works very well for anal sex because you can reach your clit with your fingers or with a small vibe while in this position. Another option is lying on your back with your legs raised. The benefit of this position is that your partner can see your face as he penetrates you. The side-by-side position, with your partner behind you, also works well. You will need to relax as you allow him to penetrate you. If you feel nervous or reluctant, you won't enjoy the sensation. Don't force anything. If you aren't enjoying it, stop and switch to another activity and try again later.

If he's taking his time and it's feeling good, he can continue to press forward until he's fully inside you. Once he is, pause for a moment and revel in the sensation of being filled in such an intimate way. When you are ready, he can start an in-and-out motion. Touch your clitoris if you want to have an orgasm this way.

Cleanliness

First of all, relax. We all have a butt, and yours is not dirtier than anyone else's. Anal sex doesn't require any special cleaning rituals, but if you want to, you can take some extra precautions to make sure you don't encounter any mess. And if you do, don't freak out. You, your partner, and your sheets are all washable. Many, many, many couples enjoy anal sex and sometimes, well, shit happens. I promise it's not a big deal.

A nice hot shower with lots of soap will get you plenty clean, but if you really want to go the extra mile, you can buy a bulb syringe at a drugstore. These look a little like turkey basters and can be found in the enema section. Fill the syringe with water, give your tush a little squirt, and let the water run out into the toilet. Do this once or twice, and you'll be all clean.

Even committed couples who don't use condoms during vaginal sex should use them for anal sex. Once he's been in your ass, he shouldn't penetrate you vaginally. Bacteria from your ass can give you a urinary tract infection or bacterial vaginosis. Using a condom solves this problem, as you can just take the condom off and throw it away. For this same reason, you should use condoms on any sex toys you use for anal penetration.

STRAP-ON SEX

Strap-on sex is not just practiced by women who have sex with women. In recent years, it's become common in couples of all varieties. There are many reasons to wear a strap-on, the most obvious being that doing so expands your sexual possibilities. For women who sleep with women, a strap-on can allow them to penetrate their partner in new, exciting ways while also leaving their hands free. Many men enjoy being penetrated anally with a strap-on as well, and adding this activity to your repertoire can inject your sex life with a very high level of excitement. A strap-on allows you to play with gender in ways you may never have done before. It also allows you to play with power and domination while augmenting your role-playing scenarios. At the least, there are certainly no downsides to giving it a try, and you may discover something you and your partner both find extremely hot.

You'll find tips for choosing a dildo and harness in chapter 11. If you don't have a reputable retailer in your town, buy your toys online. There are many, many online retailers to choose from. My personal favorites are ComeAsYouAre.com and Babeland.com. If you are buying a strap-on for the first time, choose a starter kit. It will come with a comfortable harness and a small, smooth dildo. Wearing it may feel awkward at first, though your excitement will probably temper the awkward feelings.

You may notice in the beginning that wearing a strap-on throws off your balance. If you've always been a receptive partner, thinking of your pelvis in this new way takes some getting used to. If you feel silly, go with it. Don't be shy—play around with your new cock, wear it around the house, do the dishes in it if you must. Everyone feels awkward at first. Don't worry. Wear it until it begins to feels like a part of you.

The positions described above all apply to both strap-on penetration and penis-in-vagina intercourse. Prepare your partner for anal or vaginal penetration with your strap-on in the same way you would want your lover to prepare you. Warm him or her up with foreplay and oral sex, and if you are penetrating your partner anally, use your fingers first to help him or her relax and open up. One thing to keep in mind: A silicone dildo is likely to be firmer than a penis, and women who are used to deep, hard penetration during sex with a male partner may find that the same force is too much with a dildo. As with everything, start slowly, experiment, play around, letting your partner dictate the speed and depth of your thrusts, until you find a rhythm that feels good.

If your male partner wants to be penetrated anally, you should choose the dildo together. Dildos come in every size, from pinky finger to traffic cone. I guarantee your eyes will be bigger than his ass. Always buy silicone dildos. Silicone is slightly more expensive than jelly and other rubber dildos, but those cheaper rubbers are not sterilizable. Your harness should fit snugly. Some harnesses come with a compartment that can hold a vibrator, offering more sensation for the wearer.

Wearing a strap-on dick is exciting, makes you feel powerful, and allows you to step away from the idea that women are naturally the receptive partner. Some strap-on wearers learn to create a mind-body connection and embrace their "psychic cock." You can practice connecting to your dildo in this way by asking your partner to give you a blow job while you wear it. Don't knock this until you've tried it—you'll be surprised at the amount of sensation your brain can transmit to your genitals. The dildo may not have any nerve endings, but it sure as hell works as a powerful representation of the hard-on you have going on in your head. Embrace your dick, get comfortable with it, and you may find eventually that you can climax from penetrating your partner with it.

PRACTICE MAKES PERFECT

You don't need to have simultaneous orgasms to have great intercourse. You don't need to have orgasms at all. But hopefully the techniques we've discussed in this chapter can help you make intercourse more sexy and satisfying. Some of these techniques may be new to you, some may even be awkward. Don't be afraid to laugh. So what if you fall off the bed or make funny noises. Fitting two bodies together is never as easy as it looks. If something isn't working, just switch positions and start again!

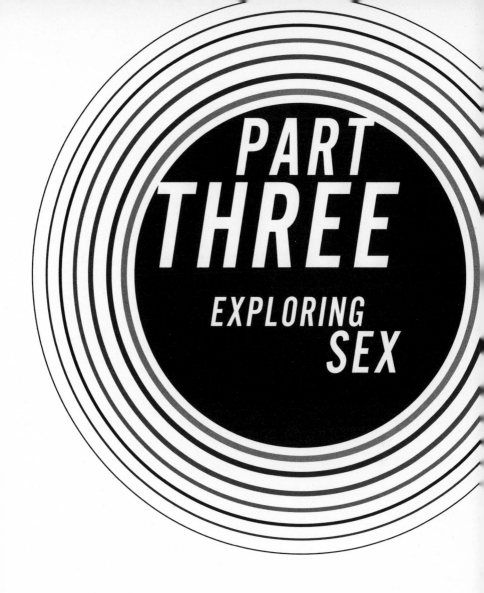

PART THREE

EXPLORING SEX

TOYS, LUBE, AND OTHER ACCOUTREMENTS

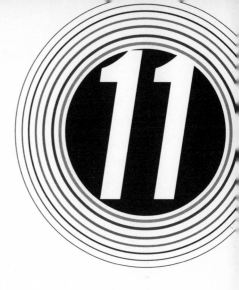

S EX TOYS ADD variety to your sex life, keep you entertained on solo nights, and help you create more satisfying erotic experiences with your partner. Toys help you take ownership of your pleasure, which in turn helps increase your overall sense of satisfaction. Introducing a sex toy is an easy way to add something new to your sex life, make sex more interesting, and help you reach orgasm more easily. Plus, the sense of sexual autonomy that comes from wielding a good sex toy leaves you feeling more self-assured and sexy and even more irresistible to your lovers. I can't think of any reason why a woman wouldn't want to own sex toys.

In case you were wondering, sex toys have been around forever—certainly long before *Sex and the City* turned everyone on to the Rabbit Vibrator. In fact, the earliest sex toy on record is the Hohle Fels phallus, a prehistoric dildo that dates back to 28,000 BCE. Interestingly, carved stone phalluses turn up relatively often on archaeological digs; according to archaeologist Timothy Taylor in *The Prehistory of Sex: Four Million Years of Human Sexual Culture,* it's apparently been the norm for archaeologists to find these carefully polished, obviously phallic-shaped "batons" and label them flint-making tools or give them some other innocuous purpose, even though they are often covered in explicit erotic symbolism. Archaeology is apparently somewhat uptight—go figure.

Around 500 BCE, we begin to find Greek vase art of images of women holding *oblisbos,* a.k.a. dildos. There are references to *oblisbos* in Greek literature; Sappho makes reference to them a couple of times, and they make an appearance in Aristophanes's play *Lysistrata.* Dildos were seemingly very popular in ancient Greece and Rome, and Pompeii is full of erotic relics. With all these dildos, folks needed lube, of course, and around 350 BCE we get the first mention of olive oil being used as a sexual lubricant.

A couple of hundred years later, we find a reference to a penis sleeve in the *Kama Sutra.* It was essentially a dildo that fits over a man's own dick to make it longer and thicker. From that point on, we start seeing all types of sex toys in Asia. Ben Wa balls, for instance, were first mentioned in 500 CE. These little metal balls—at first a single ball, and later a pair—were popular with geisha, who inserted them before intercourse to make sex more pleasurable.

Cock rings make their first appearance in 1,200 CE China. The first documented ones were made from the eyelids of goats. Men tied them around their hard-ons, goat eyelashes and all. Later in China, we find much improved cock rings, carved of ivory and jade, with ornate dragonhead designs. The carved dragon tongues formed a clit-stimulating nub, designed to increase female pleasure during intercourse.

Kinky sex shows up in about 1,750, when brothels began adding spanking, flagellation, and other SM fun to their menus. You can thank the Marquis de Sade for taking kinky sex mainstream. After the publication of his famous novel *Justine,* regular folks began to embrace riding crops, nipple clamps, restraints, and other BDSM accoutrements. The Victorians tried, of course, to clamp down on masturbation and adultery with chastity belts and other antisex devices, but engineering, sex-minded folks often took the antimasturbation designs and turned them into sex-play devices.

Vibrators appear on the scene in the late 1800s. At first they were a doctor's tool, as Rachel Maines explains in her amazing book *The Technology of Orgasm.* Doctors had been masturbating their female patients to orgasm dating all the way back to Hippocrates. (That's around 300 BCE, for those who are a little fuzzy on historical time lines.) Disturbing, isn't it, that we've been outsourcing our orgasms for several thousand years?

Designed as a treatment for hysteria, the vulvular massage treatment necessary to produce orgasm was very time-consuming when performed by hand. Vibrators significantly hurried the process along, increasing the number of patients a doctor could treat in a working day. Since hysteria was a disease that could be treated but not cured, patients had to visit their doctors on a regular basis for treatments, so, as you can imagine, the costs added up. This led to the creation of a home version of the vibrator, and in the early 1900s we began to see advertisements for handheld massagers—purported to promote vitality and health—in the back of women's magazines.

Luckily for us, vibrators have continued to evolve from the first steam-powered doctor's office apparatus in 1869 to the hand-held Vibratelle in 1899. The newest thing on the market today is a series of couple-oriented vibrators by a company called Lelo. These high-tech sex toys incorporate the same technology used in the Wii. Imagine the fun you could have with those.

CHOOSING SEX TOYS

There really are no drawbacks to incorporating sex toys into your love life. You can't become dependent on them, and they can't replace your partner. In fact, it's just the opposite: Couples who try new things together experience increased intimacy and develop deeper bonds. Sex toys can help you have a more satisfying, more exciting relationship with your lover. For some women, sex toys are occasional treats, something new to stave off boredom. For others, sex toys are more of a staple, a regular ingredient in their sex life.

Sex toys can also work like an insurance policy: If you sometimes have trouble reaching orgasm, having a vibrator at the ready can help you have worry-free sex with your partner. The two of you can go at it in whatever combination you desire, and you'll know that once you climb down from the chandelier, an orgasm awaits you.

Sex toys are sold practically everywhere now. Feminist-run sex-toy shops still represent sex-toy-shopping utopia, but major retailer chains are also in the orgasm biz. See what I mean? If we weren't meant to own sex toys, they wouldn't sell vibrators—excuse me, back massagers—at the mall. If you haven't bought sex toys before, start with something basic. You'll have plenty of time to build your collection, and while ten-inch dildos are certainly compelling, a small vibrator to stimulate the clit during intercourse should be everyone's first toy purchase.

Modern sex toys are very advanced, and many are designed for couples to use together. Today's toys incorporate new technology with cutting-edge design. If you haven't kept up with the industry, I bet you'll be blown away. Shopping for sex toys together is great fun and gives couples an excuse to be a little naughty together in public. So why not suggest a little toy shopping to your partner? Don't worry if you feel a bit awkward at first; once you've broached the subject, you'll probably find it very exciting to talk about. Sometimes, faking a little nonchalance can help you get past your nervousness. Once you've started the discussion, your nonchalance is likely to rub off on your partner, and the next thing you know, the two of you will be shopping for butt plugs with your leftover holiday gift cards.

YOUR TOY COLLECTION

Your toy chest can contain just the basics, or it can be an entire rec room full of fun. There are toys designed for you, toys designed for him, and toys designed for you to use together. Sex toys are not weird or kinky; they're fun and fabulous. Sure, it's possible to have great sex without sex toys; it's also possible to put together a great outfit without accessories. But that doesn't mean you should.

You can store your collection of accoutrements anywhere you like: A trunk at the foot of the bed, a box beneath it, and a nightstand with a good-size drawer all work well. If you have children, perhaps you'll want a drawer that locks. There are other, more decorative storage options, too. I've seen sex essentials kept in a vintage train case and an antique wardrobe next to the bed.

THE NIGHTSTAND

There are a few things you should always have within easy reach. One is a smallish vibrator you can use during intercourse. If you have multiple partners, single-use vibrating cock rings are great. You should also have safer-sex supplies, such as condoms and GLYDE dams, latex gloves, and lube. Any lube is fine, but it's nice to have a choice. I prefer a thicker lube for activities where you want a little extra cushioning, like anal play or fisting, and a thinner, more watery one for other activities. It's also nice to have massage oil, silicone lube, and hand towels nearby.

Other treats you might keep within reach include a smutty book of some kind. This could be anything from a favorite erotic novel with the steamy passages dog-eared to an anthology of erotic stories to a J/O book from the porn store. Having something smutty to read aloud is a good yet subtle way to get yourself and your partner in the mood. You can offer to read to your lover as a special bedtime treat. It may put you both in the mood, or it may simply be a nice way to relax and fall asleep. You'll also want a few candles for impromptu ambient lighting. I also keep a few scarves in the nightstand; they make great blindfolds and can be used in a pinch to tie someone up.

HOW TO CHOOSE SEX TOYS

When putting together a sex-toy collection, you'll want to consider what types of stimulation you like, what feels good, how you like to get off, and what types of things you might want to do with your partner. Do your research online; read up on toy designs, makes, and models. Figure out whether you want something for yourself, something to use with a lover, or something to use on your lover. I like ComeAsYouAre.com and Babeland.com for sex-toy shopping. Both sites are packed with reliable information, and their offerings are carefully curated by a knowledgeable staff.

VIBRATORS

Vibrators are like tireless little orgasm soldiers. There are many varieties, some designed for internal use and some only for external. There are far too many sex-toy designs to discuss them all, but we can take a tour of some of the basic models.

Tips on Choosing a Vibrator

Vibrators come in many shapes and sizes, each with its own pros and cons. Choosing a vibe you'll love takes a little thought, but don't worry—you can always buy more than one!

Jack Lamon, co-owner of the sex-toy shop Come As You Are, suggests considering these questions when choosing a new vibe:

1. Do you want a battery-powered or electric vibrator?

2. What kind of vibration are you looking for?

3. What material should your vibrator be made from?

4. How loud is your vibrator?

5. Do you want a vibrator for you, your partner, or both of you?

BATTERY-POWERED OR ELECTRIC

Battery-operated vibrators are portable and cheaper, and come in all shapes, sizes, and colors. You could buy a battery-powered vibrator to match literally every outfit you own. The drawback is that this type tends to break down more quickly than electric vibrators.

Electric vibrators are generally better made, will last for years, and provide a stronger buzz. Some need to be plugged in, but others, like several models made by Lelo and Fun Factory, are rechargeable and less bulky.

One way to narrow down your choices is to decide how you would like to use it. Ask yourself:

1. Do you want a vibrator strictly for external stimulation?

2. Will you be using it during intercourse?

3. Would you like to use it for penetration and G-spot play?

∘ *Plug-in Vibes* ∘

Plug-in vibrators, like the Hitachi Magic Wand, offer a strong, steady vibration and two basic settings (throb and jackhammer). The Hitachi is widely considered the Cadillac of vibrators, and if you've never had an orgasm, then sister, go and invest in one of these babies. Orgasms await you.

There are several versions of the Hitachi Magic Wand–style vibrator. Some are rechargeable, so you don't have to be tethered to the wall. Some are smaller and lighter, which is nice, since the Hitachi is a major appliance. It's actually a bit like having your orgasms powered by an upright kitchen mixer. Just go to the home electronics store in the mall and try them all out till you find one you like. Over your clothes, silly! You don't want to get carted off by security.

Another form of plug-in vibe is the coil-operated model. The Wahl 8-in-1 is an example of this type of vibrator. Coil-operated vibes offer a super-intense buzz and a very focused point of contact. And they are very, very quiet—so quiet, you can jerk off while your roommate is home and not have to worry about a thing. This type of vibrator is durable and very long lasting. I had one for fifteen years—that means it lasted through one marriage, one divorce, and two live-in girlfriends. I finally threw it out because I was sick of moving it from apartment to apartment.

Coil-operated vibes come with lots of attachments, and many outside companies make even more attachments that fit them. This type of vibe, like other plug-ins, usually offers only two speeds, but its steady, unwavering, strong vibrations provide effortless orgasms.

○ Rechargeable and Battery-Operated Vibes ○

Rechargeable and battery-operated vibrators come in all shapes, sizes, and colors as well. They are usually less intense than plug-in vibrators, but on the upside, they are smaller, lighter, and portable. Rechargeable vibrators are a bit pricier, but the designs are better than ever. Lelo makes wonderful high-tech vibes that last as long as seven hours off a single charge.

For the most part, battery-operated vibrators are louder than other varieties. This is because the motor and the batteries themselves are rattling around inside a plastic casing. But fear not! Several companies have caught on to the fact that we don't necessarily want the neighbors to know every time we bust out our special plastic friend, and are making battery-operated vibrators from silicones that muffle the sound quite well. Ask about the noise factor before you purchase a battery-operated vibrator, as noisy vibrators are a turnoff even when privacy isn't an issue.

DILDOS

Dildos are sex toys designed for vaginal or anal penetration. Dildos are mainly nonvibrating, come in all shapes and sizes, and are made of all sorts of materials, though I recommend buying silicone, which is stable and inert. Silicone cocks last forever. You can boil them, stick them in the dishwasher, bleach them, and wash them with soap and water. Silicone is also nonporous, so germs can't hide out and multiply.

So, what size willy do you want? I can't really answer that question for you, but I can offer up a few tips that might help you make a decision. First of all, if you are buying a dildo to use on your partner, you will probably be tempted to buy a gigantor monster dick. Because, of course, everyone wants a big dick, right? Well, she might like that, but chances are, she won't really be able to do much with it beyond admiring it from afar. Go for a more moderate size and get a bigger one later if you both agree that you want that. If you are buying it for yourself, the same thing applies. Your eyes are likely bigger than your various holes, so start small—especially if you want to use the dildo anally. If you are looking for a dildo for butt play, then start really, really small and move up as you get more relaxed.

If you think you may ever want to use your dildo in a strap-on harness, it's best to start with something that's harness compatible. This means choosing a dildo with a flared base wide enough that it won't slip through a standard harness. You'll also want to choose a dildo firm enough to fuck with. If it's too long and floppy, well, I'm sure you can imagine how it might not work out.

Double dildos allow you to enjoy the feeling of penetration while also penetrating your partner. You can use a double dildo with a partner of any gender; they aren't just for lesbian sex. Choosing the right shape and size is probably the most important part of choosing the right double dildo. Some dildos will have different-size ends, which is useful if you and your partner have different tastes. The main thing you'll need to decide is whether you want a curved or straight tool. A straight double dildo is versatile, though most people prefer the curved style because it allows for greater physical contact and more appealing positions.

NIPPLE THINGYS

Do you like to have your nipples played with? Then go get yourself a set of nipple clamps. Nipple clamps make you feel all sexy and kinky, and the sensation is fantastic. Nipple clamps come in all sorts of varieties: vibrating ones, weighted ones, ones with teeth, ones that hurt, and ones that don't. Your main goal when buying a set of nipple clamps is to make sure you don't buy some that clamp so tightly you can't bear it. Adjustable ones are a good way to go. And clothespins make a great set of nipple clamps, so you may want to start out playing with those and then move on up to something shiny and metal.

BUTT TOYS

We can all have fun with our butts. Butt play isn't weird or kinky. It's not unhealthy for you and won't cause you weird problems. It can't make a straight man gay. It doesn't make you a perv, unless you want to stick a watermelon or a cocker spaniel in there. Your butt is an equal-opportunity orifice that can be enjoyed by anyone of any gender and sexual orientation.

EXTRA CREDIT ASSIGNMENT

To learn more about safe, fun anal sex, read *The Ultimate Guide to Anal Sex for Women,* by Tristan Taormino, and *The Ultimate Guide to Anal Sex for Men,* by Bill Brent.

Technically, you can have anal sex with dildos and other types of toys, but toys designed for anal sex offer a safe way to play and are intended specifically to maximize the delicious sensation of anal penetration. If you are new to anal play, butt plugs are a good place to start. Start with the smallest plug you can find. If you end up loving it and want something bigger, you can always go get another one. But there's nothing more disappointing than buying a new toy that you can't use.

When using your butt plug, start slowly. Don't try to force it in. Press it against your butthole and relax, breathe, and bear down just a bit, until you can feel your sphincter muscles relax. When you are ready, it should slip in. Once you've got it inside, you can play around with slipping it in and out. As you get hotter and more relaxed, you'll be able to push it in farther, until you get to the point where it's in all the way and your sphincter muscles are around the neck of the plug.

Try wearing a butt plug during solo masturbation or during intercourse with your partner. The sight of the butt plug will be very exciting to your lover, and the feeling of being filled up completely will be very intense for you.

Anal beads are another fun butt-play option. These are a series of plastic beads attached to a string. You push them in and then pop them out one by one. The cheap plastic ones aren't really washable, so using them more than once is likely a no-no. But there are lots of anal beadlike options that are made of silicone. Some are simply anal beads dipped in silicone, and others are more like a long stick of silicone that has bloops of graduated sizes along the shaft.

GLASS AND METAL TOYS

Some of my very favorite insertable toys are made of glass and stainless steel. Toys made of these materials often look like works of art. The benefit to these materials is that they are extremely firm and nonporous so that lube lasts extra long. In addition, the heavy weight of metal and glass toys offers interesting and intensely orgasmic sensations that you can't really get from anything else.

Glass, acrylic, and metal toys are often a sizable financial investment, though, so unless you really fall in love with something, these are probably not going to be the first additions to your toy chest. Glass toys are made by a variety of companies but are all roughly similar. So if you are interested in glass, you'll probably have many options to choose from. The coolest stainless-steel toys are made by a company called Njoy, which offers a really beautiful selection, and the weight and shape of these toys make them powerful G-spot stimulators.

STRAP-ON HARNESSES

Strap-ons, also called strap-on harnesses or dildo harnesses, let you play with dildos while leaving your hands free for other fun. Strap-on harnesses come in several styles, from the traditional two-strap jock design to spandex shorts, G-string, corset-style, and beyond. Harnesses are made from many types of material. Leather is always popular for its durability and enduring style, though other materials also have their benefits. Nylon harnesses are cheap and versatile and great for those just starting out with strap-on play. Some strap-ons have a permanent hole for the dildo, while other designs use removable and interchangeable O-rings. The benefit of a removable ring is that you can change it out for very large or very small dildos. If you plan to use your harness with several different dildos, look for a removable O-ring. Jack Lamon suggests considering these questions before choosing a strap-on:

1. Do you want to wear it around your waist or your thigh?

2. Do you prefer a one- or two-strap style?

3. Do you need a removable O-ring?

4. Does the style you've chosen fit your body comfortably?

5. Do you feel sexy in it?

MEN'S TOYS

While most sex toys can be enjoyed by everyone, some are designed specifically with men in mind. If your male partner wants some sex toys to call his own, try indulging him with a prostate massager, a masturbation sleeve, or cock rings. Many cock rings come with vibration, which can be fun for the two of you to use together.

SEX FURNITURE

Yes, sex furniture! A company called Liberator makes excellent sex props, ramps, wedges, and even furniture designed specially for sex. These sex props improve your range of motion during any type of sex and make most positions much more comfortable. The incline these sex props offer allows deeper penetration and increased G-spot contact during intercourse in just about any position. Sex props and sex furniture can also improve oral sex and make anal sex more comfortable. Some props include built-in attachments for fun with light bondage and playful restraint.

LUBRICANTS

Lubricants make every kind of sex better—even things you thought couldn't get better. You want to use it. Lubes provide comfort and slickness, increase sensitivity, and allow you to do more things more often. Lubricants are essential for nearly all types of sex, but especially for use with sex toys and anal sex. The truth is, you will likely want to keep several types of lube around, as different formulations work better for different things.

While there are many different brands of lube, there are really only a few basic variations on lube formulas. Water-based lubricants are the most common, as they are compatible with condoms/latex and silicone toys and are easiest to clean up. Oil-based lubes are great for hand jobs and massage but will break down condoms and are generally not recommended for internal use, because it's hard for the body to flush them out. Silicone-based lubes are my personal favorite because they are long lasting and safe to use internally, although they can be harder to wash off and are more expensive. If you are interested in trying a few brands, most sex-toy retailers offer lube sampler packs containing either packets or trial-size versions of several different lubes.

Ingredients

If you are sensitive to chemicals, you should probably avoid lubes that contain nonoxynol-9 and glycerin, a contraceptive gel ingredient that most people find very irritating. Glycerin is a form of sugar. It's what makes some lubes taste sweet. Some women find that using glycerin-based lubes cause yeast infections, so if you are generally prone to yeast infections, skip these lubes.

Thicker lubes work best for anal play because they offer a little extra cushioning. Thinner lubes are good for vaginal play because they feel more similar to natural vaginal fluids. Silicone-based lubes are also popular for anal play, as they stay slick longer and are not sticky or tacky. Silicone lubes are latex-compatible and even stay slick in water, which is handy for fun in the bath or hot tub. Don't use silicone lubes on silicone or cyberskin dildos—it'll ruin them. Use a condom to prevent damaging your silicone toys with silicone lube.

THE TSA AND YOUR SEX TOYS

Traveling with sex toys has gotten a little trickier in these times of tough airport security. Every seasoned security officer has seen his or her fair share of "massagers," but it doesn't mean they won't stop and question you about an item if they can't ascertain its use. I nearly missed my flight coming back from a sex-toy convention in Las Vegas because the stainless-steel double dildo I was carrying freaked out the security staff. I had to say, "It's a sex toy; do you want me to show you how it works?" to four different people before they let me on the flight.

Know Your Rights

Security guards aren't allowed to say anything about your personal items or make you feel uncomfortable in any way. Most of them will be more embarrassed than you are about your butt-plug, so if you really love it, don't be shy about bringing it along. So what if they find it? It will tell the TSA you are a happy, sex-positive person, and that's a great thing to be.

When in Doubt, Check It

Rule number one to flying with sex toys is: Don't pack anything suspicious-looking in your carry-on; TSA guidelines are subjective at best. I once traveled from New York to Australia and back, with a stopover in Los Angeles, and didn't realize until I unpacked my bag back home in New York that I'd had a Swiss Army knife in my carry-on the entire time. No one batted an eye at the knife, but I was forced to surrender my deep conditioner in Los Angeles and spent ten days in Tasmania with split ends.

Even if you feel totally comfortable talking to the security guard and x-ray tech about your metal cock cage, carrying it onboard means a surefire bag search, and if the agent is feeling particularly unforgiving that day, you could end up being forced to check your bag at the last minute, which is annoying, to say the least.

Pack Wisely

Random searches of checked bags are routine. Expect yours to be inspected, and pack accordingly. Got something interesting in your bag? Put it in plain sight. This cuts down on the amount of time the guards will spend rifling through your tampons.

Expose Yourself to Art

Many beautiful glass, acrylic, and metal sex pieces out there double easily as a work of art. If you blanch at the idea of explaining your G-spotter to a red-faced x-ray tech, tell him or her it's a sculpture and you are a collector.

Travel Light

There's really no need to pack your Hitachi when a Pocket Rocket works just as well and takes up less space. There are also many incognito vibrators on the market, quite a few of which would fool your mom. And don't forget to remove the batteries from everything—you don't want to explain the vibrating thing in your knapsack to Grandma!

When in Doubt, Ship

I once had a disgruntled ex ship all my sex toys back to me via UPS. And while I don't recommend this as a breakup strategy, it's not a bad way to deal with sending kinky equipment. If you are going on a long trip and want to set up a sex haven at your destination, ship your equipment via UPS Ground. It will get there safe and sound just a few days after you do.

DIY Dungeons

If shipping is too much work, get creative. When you arrive at your destination, go straight to the local Home Depot for ropes and chains, hit a medical-supply store for sharp objects, and head to the grocery store for a couple of rolls of Saran wrap.

ACTING OUT
FANTASIES

12

$\mathbb{S}$ USTAINABLE, EXCITING SEX takes creativity. Or maybe it's better to say that creativity leads to sustainable, exciting sex. Either way, fantasy sex is creative, thinking sex. With a little imagination you can create unpredictable, arousing scenarios that involve seduction, fear, intimacy, violence, and taboo. Acting out fantasies lets you re-create the feeling of pursuing and being pursued. Fantasy sex can involve bondage, role-play, multiple partners, domination and submission, or not. It can also involve simple playful sex games and sexual bargaining with your lover. Certainly, building a dungeon in your basement can keep things interesting, but so can offering to submit to your partner's sexual whims in exchange for a back rub or a routine household chore.

ROLE-PLAY AND EROTIC PERSONAS

Erotic role-play is one form of acting out fantasies. It's a great way to bring a little creativity into sex play, and because erotic role-play often involves really recognizable tropes, the two of you can jump into a scenario without props or a lot of preplanning.

Erotic role-play allows you to play with overt or subtle themes of domination and submission, or act out really crazy fantasies that could never happen in reality. You can start an erotic role-play by simply adopting a well-worn script, like doctor and nurse, teacher and student, cop and robber. It doesn't have to be involved, and you don't need to act out an entire scene unless you are moved to do so. You'll probably each gravitate naturally toward the role that turns you on. That's the great thing about role-playing—it's totally up to you, and you can make your scenarios as involved or as laid-back as you like.

Don't worry about feeling silly. If you do feel silly, laugh. Crack up. Giggle. Who cares if you say something dorky? Just relax and let your inner drama geek come out. We're all a little scarred from watching too much Cinemax After Dark, but don't worry—you are far sexier and smarter than the writers who created the stock characters that are so popular in mainstream soft-core erotica. And if that type of cheesy dialogue pops into your head, take control and have some fun with it. Just because you're being sexy doesn't mean you have to drop your sense of irony.

Start with banter or an easy-to-recognize line of dialogue. For instance, if you have a particular fantasy role in mind, start by saying something that your character would say. Let's say you and your partner are fooling around in the kitchen, when you decide to start a role-play about a humorless highway patrol officer and a driver caught speeding. You could start the scene by saying coyly, "Oh, officer, I don't want to get a ticket. What can I do to convince you?" It's a recognizable script, and your partner will likely take the bait. The two of you can keep up the dialogue and roles as long as it suits you. Keep talking until you get to the bedroom; then you can choose to either drop the act when things get more serious or keep it up for the rest of the night.

One of the great things about playing this way is that it frees you to be someone else. Because you are in character, you can act out a role that the "real you" would never feel comfortable doing. Your character can be cruel and dominating, seductive and manipulating, meek and submissive, or absolutely anything you like. The "real you" might not feel comfortable acting overtly sexual, but the character you are playing certainly does.

ROLE-PLAY SCENARIOS

Get weird. Try pretending to be Lady Gaga and Katy Perry, or Terry Richardson and an American Apparel model. Bob Fosse and a horny chorus girl is a good one, too. Or stick with a classic, like a mean prison warden and a new inmate. My lover once woke me up on Easter morning and started an impromptu scene between Jesus and Mary Magdalene. Her benevolent eyes gazed lustfully at my tempting body, and we had hot sex like only a messiah and a Roman hooker know how.

Role-play gives your sex life endless opportunities for new, fun sexual scenarios. And it means you'll never get bored with your lover, since he or she can essentially become a new person whenever you want. Playing this way involves a little suspension of disbelief, but what part of sex doesn't? The best way to get into it is to keep your sense of humor. Relax and have fun and pick roles based on the sexual dynamic you are looking for. Don't agree to play slave boy if you don't want to get tied up. And if you don't want to be in charge, then angry boss isn't the right role for you.

Use props. Dress the part. I like to keep a box of costumes around for impromptu cop-and-robber scenes and trucker gang bangs, because you just never know when you might want that kind of thing. Think of role-play as a Halloween party for your bedroom. You know how Halloween is just an excuse for the popular girls to dress like prostitutes? Well, role-playing games allow you to don bunny ears and fishnets whenever the mood strikes.

Here are a few ideas to get you started:

- Pirate captain and fair maiden
- Model and photographer
- Kidnapper and hostage
- Bank robber and teller
- Slut and biker
- Priest and choir boy
- Grocery boy and soccer mom
- Mrs. Robinson and the Graduate

A NEW YOU

Sometimes you don't need an entire role-play scenario; you just want to try on a new personality for a few hours. Pretending to be someone else gives you an excuse to act outrageously and try on new things you'd otherwise be too shy to do. Your erotic persona gives you license to seduce your lover, to dress provocatively, to say things you'd normally never say. You can adopt a new personality as an experiment, use it as a way to start a conversation with a lover, or test it out just for fun and to see where it takes you. Your erotic persona can be serious, you can play at being a braver, more adventurous version of yourself, or you can adopt a character role and really try out some erotic acting. You never know where the role might take you. Here are a few to try out.

The Sex Kitten

- Turn-ons: marabou-trimmed mules, crotchless panties, soft things

- Turnoffs: working, not having sex, harsh lighting

- Icon: Elke Sommer

- Scenario: You give your sweetie a lap dance to an entire Antônio Carlos Jobim album.

The Corporate Raider

- Turn-ons: IPOs, vulnerability in others, shoulder pads

- Turnoffs: co-ops, casual Fridays

- Icon: Sigourney Weaver in *Working Girl*

- Scenario: After negotiating a successful hostile takeover, you reward your young executive assistant with a weekend in Aspen.

The Earth Mother

- Turn-ons: Gaia, eco-sexuality, chai

- Turnoffs: restrictive clothing, landfills, GMOs
- Icon: *Venus von Willendorf*
- Scenario: You and the new instructor engage in a little after hours downward dog at the yoga co-op

The Neocon Darling

- Turn-ons: Abstinence-only sex ed, the NRA
- Turnoffs: the NEA, PETA
- Icon: Ann Coulter
- Scenario: You meet a handsome stranger at an RNC fundraiser and bond while denying climate change.

The English Professor

- Turn-ons: rose gardens, the eighteenth century
- Turnoffs: bad grammar, texting
- Icon: Sally Kellerman in *Back to School*
- Scenario: Tie your lover's arms to the bedposts and read aloud from *Ulysses*.

The Artist's Model

- Turn-ons: red wine, Gauloises, the smell of turpentine

- Turnoffs: Mondrian, small talk

- Icon: Camille Claudel

- Scenario: After acknowledging your love-hate relationship, you have orgiastic sex with a brutish sculptor at the art students' ball at Place Pigalle

The Sex Nerd

- Turn-ons: Rabbit Vibrators, kneesocks, the *Kama Sutra*

- Turnoffs: sexual repression, missionary position, slut shaming

- Icon: Carol Queen

- Scenario: You and your sweetie have public sex after attending an anal-sex workshop at your local feminist sex-toy store.

TALKING, WRITING, TEXTING

Talking dirty in bed can turn run-of-the-mill sex into the hottest sex in the world. In the same vein, dirty text messages and emails are delicious foreplay. Oh my god, especially dirty text messages. It's all about the medium. Texts are short, so you have to get right to the point. And they always show up at awkward times. That's the best part. If you've ever been having lunch with your friends and gotten a text from your lover that says, "I want to fuck you right now," then you know what I'm talking about. It's like having public sex.

It can be embarrassing to talk in porno-speak if you aren't used to it. But it's a total turn-on when you do it right. I know it sounds weird, but practice when you're alone. Talking dirty on the phone and having phone sex are good practice, too. Forget the elaborate scenario—it's more about the sound of certain words and the way they make you feel. You can also use dirty talk during sex as a way to get someone to do something a little harder or softer or from a different angle.

Tread carefully at first. You want to turn your lover on, not scare him or her. Using explicit language in bed can trigger your brain-body connection and up the intensity of what's going on. Sex is best when it's taking place in your head and body at the same time. If you're usually quiet, make some noise. "Oooh," "Aaahhh," and "OhMyGod" will take you pretty far, but you can also try describing what you're doing while you're doing it. Add pet names. I like baby, sugar, daddy, cupcake, lover, officer, bastard, sir, stud, cocksucker, slut, whore, or bitch. Seriously, some perfectly reasonable people think being called a dirty cock-sucking whore in bed is the most romantic thing in the world.

Don't be vague. Use slang words and choose them carefully. "Pussy" is always good. "Cunt" and "hole" work, too. (Okay, I'm not sure about "gash," but hey, if you're more advanced than I am, run with it.)

Here's a crib sheet in case you get tongue-tied. Tape it to the wall or something.

- For lady parts: pussy, cunt, snatch, hole, box

- For manly parts: prick, cock, dick, rod

- For ass: ass, crack, asshole, hole

- For boobs: tits, rack, hooters (totally kidding about
  that last one!)

- For screwing: fuck, ball, bang, shag, stick it in

- For oral sex: eat, go down on, lick me, blow me,
  head, blow job, suck it

Now, string them all together. Pick a pet name, an action term, and a body part and make a sentence. You should come up with something like "Stick it in my pussy, you slut." Just keep it down so you don't freak out your neighbors.

EMAIL

Dirty emails are the easiest tool there is for turning your lover on. You don't have to be a great writer; simply writing out what turns you both on will work wonderfully. If you have an elaborate fantasy you would like to act out, try emailing it to your lover. Use lots of detail to help your lover envision the whole scene. Use dirty words; describe what you are wearing and how you are feeling. The nice thing about a dirty email is that you can take as much time as you like to craft it.

Don't send dirty pictures in email. Just don't do it. Learn from the mistakes of others. No matter how careful you are, I promise you they'll end up on the Internet at some point. Also, if you are sending dirty emails to your sweetie, think twice about using a work email. You are trying to turn on your partner, not the entire IT department at his or her company.

STRIPPING AND SHOWING OFF

If you enjoy being looked at by your lover, you might enjoy putting on a striptease. Stripping gives you a chance to be an object of desire. If you have fantasies about teasing, torturing, and turning on a lover, then stripping is a great way to make that a reality.

You don't actually have to be a great dancer to put on a striptease. In fact, you don't even really need to be coordinated. Forget fancy dance moves, unless you already excel in that realm. Just sway to the music and concentrate on exposing yourself a little bit at a time. Pick your favorite body part to reveal first; maybe it's your breasts or maybe it's your butt. Don't worry about looking silly—I promise you, all you need is a little music and the ability to have fun with yourself to make stripping sexy for both of you.

Dim the lights! You'll be less worried about screwing up if you are dancing in a dimly lit room. You can light candles, use a dimmer switch, or get creative with a flashlight. Candles are nice because the light is flattering to almost everyone. Have your lover sit in a chair; you can use it as a prop, dance around it, or sit on his or her lap during parts of your performance.

What will you wear? Lingerie is great, of course; you can splurge and find something kinky to strip down to. If you like to play dress-up, this is a good excuse to shop for something elaborate. However, if lingerie isn't your style, you can put on a pretty naughty show by wearing a man's shirt over a G-string. Undress by slowly unbuttoning your shirt and exposing your delightful body button by button. The trick is to make every move deliberate, turning the act of unbuttoning a shirt into a piece of erotic theater. Listen, if you're confident enough, even stripping out of your work clothes can be pretty sexy.

To gain a little confidence and maybe even learn some moves, you might watch a documentary on the art of burlesque. If you search for burlesque shows on YouTube, you'll find an abundance of performances by dancers of all shapes and sizes. That's one lovely thing about the burlesque revival that's currently so popular—there are dancers of every body type you can imagine. The sexiness isn't about having a certain body type; it's about highlighting your best assets, showing off your curves, and teasing your audience into submission. It's about flaunting what you've got and leaving the rest to the imagination.

PLAYING WITH POWER

Power means everything in this world, doesn't it? I mean, as women we're especially aware of power dynamics because in our society we're often on the "less" end of the power spectrum. One of the reasons playing with power dynamics can be very sexually exciting is that it offers us a way to have control over our partners, either by submitting willingly, which is itself a form of having power, or by taking a dominant role and forcing our lover to submit to our will.

Dominance and Submission

You don't have to be a hardcore sadist or masochist to have fun with SM fantasies, nor do you need to join a community, buy outfits, or adopt a lifestyle. Certainly, you can do all of those things—if you find them exciting, I encourage you to follow your desires. But you don't have to do anything special beyond tapping into some of your erotic desires and opening your mind to new possibilities. If you want to spank your lover or receive a spanking, or if you fantasize about being tied up and brought to the brink of orgasm, there is no reason you can't bring some of that into your sex play.

You can be submissive without being a masochist. Masochists enjoy painful sensations and find them arousing, and you may like that kind of play. But it's not a requirement. You can simply be bossed around, told what to do, and forced to perform sexual acts. If you would like to play at being submissive, have your lover create a list of demands or tasks that he or she wants you to complete. The tasks can be domestic or sexual, and if it turns you on, you can even incorporate costumes. Doesn't being "forced" to vacuum the living room while naked and in nipple clamps seem a lot more exciting that boring old housework?

If you are more the dominant type, you can start with calling the shots in bed, telling your partner what to do and when to do it. A well-timed command like "turn over" is sure to have an arousing effect on both of you. When you are ready to go further, have your partner brush your hair, paint your toenails, or give you oral sex. Use a serious voice and give commands with confidence. You can get anyone to do just about anything by ordering him or her around in a stern, unwavering tone. Try it and see.

Bondage Basics

The best way to get people to give up all control is to tie them up and maybe gag them. Then what are they gonna do about it, huh? Acting out your fantasies of being tied up or of tying someone up can be extremely exciting. You can tie up your lover and masturbate while he or she watches, perform oral sex on him or her, or slowly strip and put on a show.

SAFE WORDS

In a bondage scene, "no" may sometimes mean "yes," "stop" can mean "don't stop," and "that hurts" can mean "I'm going to come." The best way to negotiate this somewhat confusing syntax problem is to designate a safe word. When someone uses the safe word, it means the scene gets stopped and everyone gets untied, no questions asked. Your safe word can be anything, but one common trick is to use "red," "yellow," and "green" to control the intensity of what you are doing. "Red" means "stop immediately"; "yellow" means "slow down, it's getting too intense"; and "green" means "I'm okay, start back up again."

SAFE RESTRAINT

Restraining someone with something you cannot easily undo is, well, stupid. Stick with things that come off easily. If you can't resist the fetishistic appeal of handcuffs, buy the fur-lined variety. If you can find the type that don't need a key, even better. Restraints that buckle are more practical and come in many varieties of lovely soft leather. Soft cotton clothesline is good, but be careful you don't tie the knots too tightly. Neckties work nicely and so do scarves, though the drawback to using scarves is that the knots can easily become very tight. Make sure to keep scissors in your nightstand in case you can't undo a knot. Never tie anything around your lover's neck.

Once you have your lover all tied up, you can have your way with him or her. You can torture him by stroking him with soft things like feathers or fur mitts. You can tease her with ice, clothespins, tickling, biting, and slapping. Or you can blindfold him and talk dirty until he begs to be released. Try teasing her with a vibrator or other sex toy. And if you are feeling very, very cruel, you can tie him up and then ignore him.

Try adding a blindfold or even earplugs. Any type of sensory deprivation will make anything you do to your partner seem that much more intense.

PLAYING WITH PUNISHMENT

Sometimes, in the middle of a fantasy or role-play, your submissive lover is very naughty and needs a good spanking. Or maybe it's you who needs the spanking but you can't figure out how to finagle your way into one. Spanking is one of those fun but slightly intimidating activities that everyone eventually embraces. I remember teaching one of my lovers to spank me. She was a good Midwestern girl and nervous about anything she thought of as vaguely kinky. So I coaxed her into it by lying facedown on the bed with my skirt pushed up. I asked her to smack my ass, and she did, and clearly enjoyed it. But—explaining she felt too silly—she couldn't take the initiative to do it on her own. I eased her into it by asking for each smack before she delivered it, and by the end of our playtime, my obvious physical excitement was enough to make her want to spank me every time we had sex.

Tips for Giving a Hot Spanking

1. Find a sex position. Bent over something is always a crowd-pleaser. Beds, couches, laps—all of these are good options.

2. Warm up. Don't just start smacking away. Start with light taps. Rub his or her cute little butt in between smacks to keep the connection.

3. Make your spanking recipient count the hits as you go. If you are really mean, you can make him or her thank you.

4. Talk a blue streak. You know how to talk dirty. Now do it. Tell your bottom what a bad boy or girl he or she is. Tell him or her exactly what you plan to do.

5. Concentrate your smacks on the fleshy part of the butt. This is safer, feels better, and sends a lot of nice reverb throughout the genitals.

6. Add some extras. Hair pulling is nice. Try it out and see. Go softly at first—you want to turn him or her on, not piss anyone off.

7. Compliment his or her ass. Tell your spankee how nice he or she looks bent over.

8. Use a paddle. I have bruised my hand on quite a few rumps. Don't let this happen to you.

9. Cool down. When you get near the end of the spanking, ask your naughty little bottom how he or she would like to cool down. He might want the taps to come more slowly, or maybe she wants them more softly.

10. Bask in the afterglow. Hug, cuddle, fuck, or do whatever it is you like to do.

ADVENTUROUS MONOGAMY

There are many ways to open up your relationship, but a three-way has got to be one of the most common fantasies out there. If you and your lover have talked about having a three-way or engaged in three-way fantasy talk, you might be ready to give it a try. Three-ways are also a way to experiment with nonmonogamy in an environment that feels safe for all parties. If you are an established couple, it's a way to explore sex with a new person and try new things but still feel together and connected. A three-way can be your entry into playing with partners outside your relationship, or it can just be a way to see your partner in a new light. For curious couples, inviting someone else into your bedroom is sure to switch up your dynamic by allowing you to explore all sorts of new roles and ideas. You'd be surprised how exciting it can be to suddenly see your lover through a fresh lens.

Three-ways are exciting. Three people can do things that two people can't. When there are more people, there are more arms and legs, hands, pussies, and penises to play with. It's a great way to indulge either your exhibitionist or voyeuristic tendencies and fantasies. For instance, have you ever fantasized about being penetrated by two people at once? Or maybe dreamed of having your bed become a tangle of arms and legs, with bodies piled on top of each other? Maybe you've wanted to experiment with BDSM or switch up your normal role by topping if you are usually on the bottom, or vice versa. A three-way is the perfect scenario in which to make this kind of thing happen.

It's also a great way to experiment with someone of the same gender if you haven't done it before. A lot of otherwise straight folks, both men and women, state that they felt more comfortable having first-time same-sex experiences when someone of the opposite sex was present.

SEX PARTIES

Play parties and sex parties are pretty much just social gatherings where people engage in sex. They take many forms—they can be elaborately themed fetish parties with over a hundred people walking around in beautiful latex and leather outfits, kind of like a horny ball, or they can be a regular old orgy where a bunch of enthusiastic people show up and get naked in the hot tub or a kiddie pool full of olive oil or wherever happens to be handy.

One way to ensure your sex-party experience is a good one is to decide what type of setting appeals most to you. A huge party might be overwhelming. On the other hand, a very large party where you don't know most of the people might offer you the anonymity you need to let go of some of your inhibitions.

Sex parties can be loads of fun. Even if you are too shy to have sex in front of lots of people, attending a sex party is a great way to join a sex-positive community and expand your network of lovers and friends. Whether or not you've had any experience with multiple-partner sex, a play party is going to introduce you to a lot of new things and help you to expand your sexual repertoire. You'll get to see new people having all different types of sex, and you might learn some tricks. If you've ever been curious about flogging, piercing, fetishes, or other kinky activities, a play party is a good place to witness these activities being performed by people who know what they're doing. And later, when you become more comfortable, it's a great place to find willing partners and try out your new tricks. I honed my spanking skills at sex parties, first by watching skilled spanking tops dish it out and later by spanking willing bottoms.

Play parties are everywhere. Asking around or checking the local papers is often all it takes to locate one. Larger parties are often held in clubs where you won't necessarily need an invite, but that may charge cover and enforce a dress code. It really depends on the town you live in and how organized the partygoing population is.

Private parties are usually invite only, and you may need to know someone who attends regularly in order to find out about them or to get on the invite list. But as long as you are polite and open-minded, there's no reason why you won't get invited. The hard part will be tracking down the party in the first place. Don't be discouraged by this—a little bit of exclusivity will make the party better.

Start at your local sex shop or porn boutique and look for flyers or local papers with classified ads. Or ask the people who work there. Chances are, if they are working at a sex shop, they are part of the sex-positive community. If you don't have any sex shops, look for an alternative newspaper or magazine at an independent bookstore; magazines often have sex-party ads in the back. If that doesn't work, head to the Internet! Get online and find a sexually oriented discussion board or a site like Craigslist .org, where people often post personal ads. Post a query about sex parties in your area and see what turns up. As is usually the case with the Internet, someone will know someone who will know someone who throws sex parties. Even the reddest of the red states have sex-positive communities. In fact, the more conservative a town, the more pervy its perverts will be.

You can attend a sex party solo or with a partner. In mixed-gender environments, single men often are required to follow certain rules that couples and single women aren't held to, mainly to encourage everyone to behave nicely. Think about it: Single women aren't going to show up at sex clubs and parties if they have to worry about getting harassed by trench coat–wearing wankers, so respect the rules and everyone will have fun.

If you are an orgy virgin, the best way to have fun at a sex party is to lower your expectations and realize that real life isn't like *La Dolce Vita* or *Caligula*. A sex party is going to be full of regular people, some of whom you will find attractive and some of whom you won't. You should always be polite, have firm boundaries, keep an open mind, and be nice to people who approach you, even if you don't want to have sex with them.

WILD AND CRAZY IS ONLY ONE OPTION

Role-playing, three-ways, sex parties, and other adventures are completely optional. You may go through your entire life having thrilling, mind-blowing monogamous sex in bed with your partner, and that's great! You don't need to engage in extracurricular activities to enjoy sex. The point of this chapter is to show you that there's an entire world of fun things to do—or not. For many of us, certain types of sex are best explored only in fantasy. Use the information in this chapter however you wish. It may lead you down an interesting path of experimentation, or simply provide fodder for fantasies and solo sex.

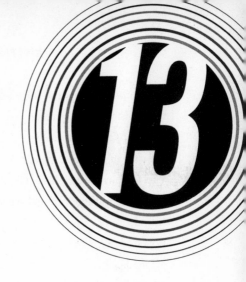

SEXUAL HEALTH AND SAFER SEX

P ART OF BEING a good lover and having a great sex life is taking care of your body, your mind, and your sexual health. Sex, like any other wonderful thing, involves risks, though, if you're equipped with the right information and precautions, they aren't that big a deal. Keep in mind that your emotional health is just as important as your physical health—they work synergistically. When we're emotionally healthy, we are more likely to take care of our physical bodies, and when our physical bodies are in good shape, we have a healthier self-image. Positive self-image has been associated with better self-care strategies, and women who feel happier with their bodies have been shown to be more likely to seek out regular gynecological care.

HEALTH IS SEXY

We think of hard-partying people as having tons of sex, but the reality is that a hard-partying lifestyle is associated with just the opposite. Danish researchers found that smoking, drinking, and drug use have been linked to poor-quality sex lives for both men and women, and that in some cases partying correlates directly to a complete lack of partner sex. The same study, published in the *Journal of Sexual Medicine,* indicated that for partnered individuals, risk of sexual dysfunction increased significantly in people who lead unhealthy lives. Drug use was linked to various types of sexual dysfunction, including lack of orgasm in women. Not only do unhealthy people have sexual problems, but the study indicated that people who are sexually inactive are more likely to engage in unhealthy behavior. So not only is being healthy good for your sex life, but a good sex life is good for your health.

LISTEN TO YOUR BODY

Healthy does not always equal thin, and thin doesn't necessarily mean healthy. Rather than waste time trying to meet a media-created body "ideal," choose to love the body you have. If your weight falls outside a healthy range—and research shows that "healthy" range is far larger than magazines would have you think—try to gently bring yourself closer to a weight that works for you. Be kind to yourself. There is no need to drastically restrict your diet unless a doctor tells you it's necessary. While many of us assume that body dissatisfaction drives us to take care of ourselves, the opposite is actually true. Researchers at Ohio State University found that women who accept themselves are more likely to make healthy food choices and take care of their bodies. Read and learn about nutrition, exercise, and fitness. Pay attention to the cues your body gives you. Eat when you are hungry; talk a walk when you feel listless. The best thing you can do for your sex life is take good care of your body.

SEXERCISE

All exercise improves mood, health, and body image, but did you know that certain exercises have significant sex benefits? Yoga, Pilates, and other forms of exercise that emphasize core strength and flexibility are great for sex. Regular exercise decreases stress levels and helps you relax and get into the mood. When your body is strong, you can go longer and harder, and upper-body strength helps you stay longer in compromising positions. Another benefit: Improved circulation means greater blood flow to the genitals. Most important, exercise improves your mood, and a happier you is a sexier you.

A HAPPY YOU

Just as important as taking care of your body with good nutrition and exercise is taking care of your emotional well-being through self-care, stress management, and seeking help when necessary. When we feel positive about our lives and good about ourselves, the quality of our sex life reflects it.

How much time do you waste thinking about the body you wish you had? Do you ever find yourself putting off enjoyable activities until after you lose weight? Instead of fantasizing about a different body, spend more time enjoying the one you have now. Sure, that's easier said than done, but start with small changes. The language we use shapes the way we think about something. Drop negative statements. Use language that makes you feel empowered. For example, "I hate my body" is very negative and leaves little room for change, whereas the statement "I'm working on myself" is a way of expressing your dissatisfaction while still empowering yourself to make changes. Think it's too simple and can't possibly work? Try consciously changing your negative statements for a week, and then see how you feel about yourself.

DITCH YOUR STRESS

We're all stressed out. We're overworked. We don't get enough sleep. And we only make it worse when we don't take enough time for ourselves. Stress kills your sex life. It prevents you from being present during sex and can even prevent you from getting in the mood. Stress chemicals age you, and stress creates havoc in your body. Make a pact with yourself to get off the twenty-four-hour stress cycle right now.

Start with some time alone. Obviously, for women with busy careers and families, alone time is hard to come by, but it doesn't need to be very long. Can you squeeze in a half hour for yourself? Explain to your partner that helping with kids and housework so that you can have time to reset will pay off for both of you. Take a bath or read. Create a ritual in which you get a half hour before bed to do whatever you like. Use your time to unplug your brain.

When we're single, it's not our lack of alone time that feels stressful; it's the occasional fear that we may have too much of it. Long evenings stretched out in front of us can feel very isolating, and it's easy to fill the time with TV and a glass (or seven) of wine. There's nothing wrong with drinking and watching TV in moderation, but too many nights like this can lead to depression. Instead of turning on the television, try connecting with friends. Make an effort to call someone. Keep your drinking to a minimum. A little alcohol can help you relax, but regular consumption can lead to a whole lot of health problems, both emotional and physical.

MASTURBATE

We've talked about masturbation throughout this book. I've suggested masturbation as a way to have orgasms during intercourse, as a way to learn about your sexual responses, and as a way to be sexual when you don't have a partner. But masturbation can also be used as a mood lifter and a stress reducer. Several studies show that it's beneficial for your overall health.

Regular masturbation makes you more resistant to yeast infections. It eases menstrual cramps and increases blood flow to the pelvic region, which helps ease back pain. It relieves stress, helps you sleep, boosts your mood, and helps you stay healthy by familiarizing you with your genitals. If you touch your pussy every day, you'll know right away if something seems wrong and you'll be able to get to the doctor before any problems become worse. Masturbation helps keep your pelvic-floor muscles in good shape, preventing urinary incontinence. It also makes you feel connected to your body, and that helps you feel powerful.

HAVE REGULAR CHECKUPS

Taking care of your gynecological health by having regular checkups—including pelvic exams, Pap smears, and breast cancer screenings—is a vitally important part of your sexual well-being. Routine visits help prevent illness and can catch problems early. If you have an abnormal Pap, for example, there are important tests and treatments available that can prevent cervical cancer. Taking care of your health is part of loving yourself.

If you feel uncomfortable seeking gynecological care, put the effort into finding a good practitioner. Many women who are queer, intersex, masculine in their gender presentation, or trans fear discrimination by health care providers and as a result don't seek regular medical care. This is tragic. Not seeking medical care because you fear prejudiced doctors lets the bigots win. Your health is important. Trans men, listen up: Even if you have had top surgery, you need to check the remaining breast tissue regularly for lumps. Even if you take testosterone, you need routine gynecological checkups. You've worked hard to get this body—now take care of it.

If a health care provider discriminates against you, shames you, or makes you uncomfortable in any way, let him or her know how you feel. If the provider continues, leave and find another one. It's awful that I have to say this, but it's even more awful that there are bigoted, misogynistic, sex-negative, homophobic health care providers out there. Don't let anyone shame you. Don't let ignorant bigots keep you from taking care of yourself. Finding a sensitive practitioner is easier than you think. If your town has no feminist health care clinic, head to the Internet for suggestions.

EMBRACE YOUR SEXUALITY

Self-knowledge and self-love are the primary ingredients in a great sex life. Explore your sexuality with your lovers. Work to overcome inhibitions and shame. Rather than worrying about the way your body looks, focus on what it can do. Enjoy every orgasm you are fortunate enough to give and receive. Enjoy the feel of your own skin and that of your lover. Take up space in the world as a sexual person. The more you enjoy yourself, the more you'll inspire all the people around you to enjoy themselves. You can create positive change just by being yourself. Think about it this way: In a world full of shame and ignorance, being a sexually happy woman is a revolutionary act.

PREGNANT SEX

Some women want sex when they're pregnant, others don't. The first trimester is full of hormonal fluctuations, nausea, and mood swings, and leaves some women feeling less than sexy. The second trimester, however, can be just the opposite. The nausea has passed, your body is changing, and you're probably starting to feel excited about being a mom. In fact, some of the physiological changes that happen during your second trimester, like swollen genitals and breasts, can leave you feeling extra interested in sex.

Sex during pregnancy is perfectly fine. As long as you are having a healthy pregnancy, there is no reason why you and your partner should not continue to be sexual when you feel like it. Pregnancy is a time when you get to really celebrate your curves and lusciousness. Some women feel especially sexy and freer in their bodies when they are pregnant, and their increased genital blood flow makes them more easily turned on and sexually responsive, and even more easily orgasmic.

You'll probably have to experiment with positions to find a way to please your changing body, but rest assured, there are no off-limits positions, I don't care what your girlfriend or boyfriend thinks—his penis or her dildo just isn't that big!

The bottom line is, if the mood strikes, go ahead and get it on during those nine months prebaby. Chances are, you won't have as many opportunities for alone time once the baby arrives, so take advantage of your last few months of private time.

BIRTH CONTROL

Being heterosexually active means you must think about birth control. Previous generations had very little control over the timing of pregnancy, and that had a tremendously negative impact on women's lives, health, and careers. Now, despite the fact that control of our reproductive rights is constantly under siege by right-wing legislators, we have more birth control options than ever before. The best way to find a method that works for you is to read up on the options and talk with a healthcare practitioner. However, there are a few things you should consider when making your choice.

1. Make a decision about birth control before you start to have sex.

2. Decide whether you want to have sole responsibility for your method of birth control or whether you want to share the responsibility with a partner.

3. Discuss with your partner whether or not you may want to become pregnant in the future.

4. Carefully consider the pros and cons of any birth control method you choose.

5. Once you've chosen a method of birth control, use it consistently.

Forms of Birth Control, in Order of Effectiveness

1. Sterilization, IUD, implant

2. The Shot, the Ring, the Pill, the Patch

3. Diaphragm, female condom, male condom, withdrawal, sponge, cervical cap

4. Spermicide, fertility awareness (rhythm method)

Keep in mind that the only method of birth control that also protects you from STDs is condoms. Even if you are on the Pill, you must use a condom for safer sex.

SEX AND AGING

There's no reason why we can't enjoy sex for as long as we want to! In fact, getting older has a few advantages. Once children leave home, you have more time alone, you don't have to worry about getting knocked up, and you've lived in your body long enough that you've finally come to accept it. Studies even show that women report higher sexual satisfaction and more frequent orgasms as they get older. Let's face it—our bodies might be smoking hot when we're younger, but we don't figure out what to do with them until we're older. No way would I go back to being twenty-one! Think about it—would you? Would you *really?*

Our aging bodies are just as capable of sexual pleasure as they were when we were young—we just need to be a little creative. We may not have the same mobility at sixty-three that we did at twenty-three, but that just means it's time to come up with new positions and techniques. There are many reasons to maintain your sex life as you get older, some of the most important being that continuing to have sex with our partners helps keep our relationships strong and happy. Also, being sexual allows us to revel in the positives of our bodies and keeps us from getting down about the inevitable changes aging brings.

The best way to keep your body primed for sex as you age is to stay active. Cardiovascular activity helps blood circulation, an important component of a sexually healthy body. One issue postmenopausal women face is the thinning of their vaginal walls due to dropping hormone levels. Low estrogen also means we have less natural lubrication. But don't worry—using a lubricant can solve this problem.

Have more sex. The more sex you have, the more likely you are to want it. Any sexual activity counts; you don't need a partner to be sexual. Make sure to masturbate! Masturbation can help your pussy stay young by helping to prevent atrophy of the vaginal walls. It also boosts your mood and makes you feel better about yourself. Try using a vibrator; it's easier on drier, more delicate tissues than fingers are.

Joan Price is an advocate for ageless sexuality and a vibrant, beautiful example of the way sex keeps us young. She's the author of two books on senior sex, *Better Than I Ever Expected: Straight*

Talk About Sex After Sixty and *Naked at Our Age: Talking Out Loud About Senior Sex*. Joan offers the following tips for hot sex after sixty. You can find more, including fantastic tips for solo sex after sixty, on her website, JoanPrice.com.

Ten Tips for Hot Sex After Sixty

1. Slo-o-o-w-w down. Yes, it takes longer to warm us up. Fortunately, one of the best things about midlife and later-life sex is the absence of urgency for our partners, also. They enjoy slow sex as much as we do! Make sex play last hours . . . or days.

2. Kiss and kiss. Kiss sweetly, passionately, quickly, slowly, contentedly, hungrily, lightly, sloppily. All kinds of kisses help you bond with your partner, warm up, and enjoy the moment.

3. Appreciate, decorate, and celebrate your own and your partner's bodies. Jewelry, lingerie, feathers, fringe, silk, velvet, massage oil, candlelight— whatever looks good feels good.

4. Do sexy things together long before you hit the sheets. Dance together. Visit lingerie or sex-toy shops. Leave sexy notes in each other's pockets. Give each other little gifts.

5. Do sexy things on your own to get yourself in the mood. Wear sexy lingerie under your everyday clothes. Work out. Swim. Dance. Fantasize. Write

in your journal all the sexy things you want to do together. Spend some time humming with your vibrator.

6. Make love during high-energy times. Midnight sex after a romantic meal may work for young folks, but we're more likely to feel full, bloated, and ready to sleep. Instead, make sex dates in the morning or afternoon. (Why do you think they call it "afternoon delight"?)

7. Explore sex toys and other erotic helpers. Our hormonally challenged bodies may need extra help to reach orgasm these days. Lucky for us that sex toys are easy to find, fun to try, and wow, do they work!

8. Use a silky lubricant. We don't have the natural moisture we used to, but there are many different lubricants that feel great and bring back the joy of friction. When your partner applies it, it becomes an erotic part of sex play.

9. Enjoy quality snuggle time before, during, and afterward. Holding each other, feeling the warmth and texture of each other's skin, is one of the sweetest and sexiest parts of making love.

10. Laugh a lot. Play silly games, invent special words, tease each other, rediscover your childhood together. Laughter is bonding, joyful, ageless—and sexy.

SAFER SEX

Most of us understand that sexual activity, especially with a new partner, carries risk. We're aware we should protect ourselves from STDs by having only safer sex; however, not all of us understand what does and what doesn't constitute safer sex. Unfortunately, the only absolutely foolproof protection against STDs is to have "no contact" sex. Phone sex and cybersex are two examples of "no contact" sex. Even manual sex carries some risk; genital warts, for instance, can be transmitted via the hands.

One form of safer sex is called "fluid bonding." If you are fluid bonded with your partner it means you have both been tested for STDs, have received a clean bill of health, and have agreed to either have no other partners or have only protected sex with other partners. Keep in mind that this form of safer sex is not foolproof, because people, even people we love, are not always honest.

Luckily, great sex is about a lot more than a penis going in a pussy or a butt. There are many exciting ways you and your partner can turn each other on that carry very little risk. Getting creative about safer sex is a great way to discover new ways of giving and receiving sexual pleasures.

Planned Parenthood categorizes the following activities as "very low risk" for the transmission of STDs:

- Fantasy, cybersex, or phone sex

- Using clean sex toys

- Masturbation or mutual masturbation

- Manual stimulation of one another

- Touching or massage

- Fondling or body rubbing

- Kissing

- Oral sex on a man with a condom

- Oral sex on a woman with a GLYDE dam or plastic wrap

Planned Parenthood categorizes the following activities as "low risk" for the transmission of STDs:

- Deep kissing that causes bleeding

- Vaginal intercourse with a condom or female condom

- Anal intercourse with a condom or female condom

- Oral sex (avoid getting semen, vaginal fluids, or blood into the mouth or on broken skin)

Planned Parenthood categorizes the following activities as "high risk" for transmitting STDs:

- Vaginal intercourse without a condom

- Anal intercourse without a condom

STDS

Sexually transmitted infections are commonly referred to as STIs or STDs. And honey, I hate to break it to you, but the world is full of them. You must learn to talk to a partner about safer sex, set sexual boundaries, and use protection to avoid transmission. If you haven't been screened for STDs recently, why not do so now? Being screened allows you to start with a clean slate by ensuring you aren't harboring an asymptomatic infection. Get tested now and then continue to do so regularly.

Talking About STDs

The safe-sex talk should be an early part of your relationship and something you revisit from time to time. Getting tested together is a smart way to begin a sexual relationship; if you go together, you can offer each other support. If you know you have an STD, it's your responsibility to discuss it with your partner before you have any sexual contact. Some people with chronic infections, like genital herpes, struggle with when to "come out" about their STD to a potential partner. You should bring it up when you feel comfortable doing so, but definitely before genital contact of any kind. Your partner may have questions and concerns, so be sure you have all the information you need to address his or her fears. Don't feel ashamed or embarrassed—STDs are simply a fact of life, and most sexually active people contract some type of sexually transmitted infection at some point. Be prepared by learning as much as you can about STDs and safer-sex methods.

Living with STDs

The most reliable method of protecting yourself and your partner from STDs is to use condoms. If one or the other of you is unsure about your STD status, you should use condoms for intercourse and oral sex, and women should use a latex dam when receiving oral sex. If you or your partner know that you have an STD, you should continue to use condoms and dams every time you have sex.

Condoms

The easiest way to protect yourself from infections and unwanted pregnancies is to use condoms every time you have sex. Infections are present in highly concentrated amounts in semen, and your vagina, mouth, and rectum are highly permeable mucus membranes. This makes unprotected intercourse and oral sex a high-risk activity for the transmission of infections. Luckily, when used correctly, condoms significantly lower your risk of transmitting infections.

To put on a condom, first remove it from its wrapper and determine which way it unrolls. Make sure it isn't inside out before placing it over the head of the penis. If your condom has a receptacle tip, squeeze it to remove the air before unrolling it. If the condom doesn't have a receptacle tip, leave a little space at the end. Putting a dab of lube on the inside of the condom before putting it on can significantly improve sensation for your male partner.

Condom fit is very important. A loose-fitting condom can slip off the penis, and a condom that fits too tightly is at risk of breaking during intercourse. Condoms come in a variety of sizes, shapes, colors, scents, and styles. Finding one that meets all your needs shouldn't be that hard.

Practice good condom etiquette. It's important that your partner grasp the base of the condom as he withdraws from your vagina; otherwise, the condom may slip off his penis. This is especially important if he has ejaculated or otherwise lost his erection. Think of it this way: Fishing around in your coochie for a stray condom is indelicate at best.

Barriers for Oral Sex

You can transmit STDs through unprotected oral sex as easily as you can through unprotected intercourse. Use a condom for performing fellatio; it will still feel good for him and will keep you both safe from infections. If you don't like the taste of latex, try using flavored condoms. Mint-flavored ones are especially awesome.

You can also make cunnilingus safer by using a latex barrier. GLYDE dams are made specifically for cunnilingus and come in many flavors. To use a dam, hold it over your partner's vulva while licking and pleasing her. If the dam slips off, switch to a fresh one so you don't accidentally mix up the pussy side with the tongue side. Plastic wrap makes a nice substitute for dams; it's thinner and see-through, and you can tear off as big a piece as you'd like.

Human Papillomavirus (HPV)

HPV is the most common STD. And by "common," I mean half of all men and more than three out of four women contract it at some point. Over one hundred strains of the virus exist, though not all are harmful. Low-risk strains of HPV can cause genital warts, and high-risk strains, if left untreated, can lead to cervical cancer, infertility, and anal cancer in men.

Most people don't know they have HPV infections, so it's important to get regular Pap smears to detect the virus and receive follow-up treatment if necessary. Most HPV infections, though not all, are cleared by the body's immune system within two years. An HPV vaccine has been approved for girls and women aged nine to twenty-six, and vaccines for other segments of the population are currently being developed.

Herpes

Herpes has no cure, and while it is not fatal, people who are infected often face symptomatic outbreaks throughout their lives. It is possible to have an asymptomatic herpes infection, but it's unlikely. Most people have at least one breakout, and most experience breakouts on a regular basis. Symptoms include painful blisters on the genitals or around the mouth. Herpes is transmitted by skin-to-skin contact; you can get oral herpes on your genitals, and vice versa. Once someone contracts herpes, he or she is always infectious, even without having any visible sores.

Syphilis

During the first stage of syphilis, an open sore, called a chancre, appears. You may have just one chancre; you may have a few. Chancres usually appear about three weeks after infection but may take up to ninety days to show up. Without treatment, they last three to six weeks. Chancres can appear on the genitals, in the vagina, or on the cervix, lips, mouth, breasts, or anus. Swollen glands may also occur during the primary phase. The second stage of syphilis includes a whole-body rash and other symptoms, including mild fever, fatigue, sore throat, hair loss, weight loss, swollen glands, headache, and muscle pains. The only way to protect yourself from syphilis is to use a condom. Untreated syphilis can cause death.

Common Bacterial Infections

Chlamydia, gonorrhea, trichomoniasis, and bacterial vaginosis are bacterial infections and can be treated with antibiotics. All of them can be transmitted through oral, anal, or vaginal sex. These infections often exhibit similar symptoms, including foul odor, discharge, pain when urinating, and vaginal itching. Many bacterial infections can lead to infertility if they are not treated. Untreated chlamydia can cause long-term problems, including pelvic inflammation, swollen or scarred fallopian tubes, and chronic pain. The only way to protect yourself from contracting these infections is to use a condom.

HIV/AIDS

HIV is the virus responsible for AIDS (acquired immune deficiency syndrome). You cannot know for sure that you don't have HIV until you get tested; about one in four people with HIV is unaware he or she is carrying the virus. If you have never been tested for HIV, you should be, even if you have no reason to think you have ever come in contact with the virus. The reality is, it's not possible to know the complete history of all of our sexual partners. There's no drawback to getting tested. You'll probably find that it feels empowering—it shows that you care about your health and the health of your partners. Getting tested is responsible.

Some women avoid getting tested for HIV because they are afraid of the results, while others find that the idea of being tested causes them such anxiety that they choose not to think about it. This reaction is understandable: Since the very beginning of the epidemic, HIV/AIDS has been more stigmatized than any other STD, mainly because it was originally linked to groups that already faced a lot of prejudice. Because the disease is spread through sexual contact, it made great fodder for politicians and religious wingnuts with a moral agenda to promote. Hypocritical moralizing and sexual shame held back AIDS research for several decades. Even now, people living with HIV face intense discrimination. To this day, there is no cure for HIV/AIDS, although recent advancements in treatment allow those diagnosed with the virus to live far longer than they did several years ago.

The best way to protect yourself from infection is to learn about the virus and use protection every time you have sex. You cannot catch HIV through casual contact like kissing or holding hands. You cannot spread HIV/AIDS through hugging, sharing towels, or drinking out of the same glass. You cannot spread HIV/AIDS by holding someone or sharing a bed.

HIV is transmitted through blood, semen, vaginal fluids, and breast milk. It is most commonly spread through unprotected vaginal or anal intercourse or through sharing needles with a person who has the virus. Babies born to women with HIV/AIDS can get HIV from their mothers during birth or from breastfeeding.

SAFE, SANE, AND RESPONSIBLE

We've covered a lot of ground in this chapter, and at the same time we've barely scratched the surface. I'm sure you realize by now that being sexually active means taking responsibility for yourself and your lover. Approach every sexual encounter seriously. Not only is your physical health at stake, but so is your emotional well-being and the emotional well-being of the person you're having sex with. Never take anyone for granted. Don't use sex as a tool to get things you want or to manipulate someone into having feelings for you. Sex is too wonderful to be treated trivially. Every sexual encounter has the potential to lead to something greater, and often that greater thing is love.

WORKS CITED

Addington, Deborah. *A Hand in the Bush: The Fine Art of Vaginal Fisting*. San Francisco: Greenery, 1997.

"Aristotle's Masterpiece: The Secrets of Nature Displayed." *The Ex-Classics Web Site*. www.exclassics.com/arist/ariscont.htm (accessed June 26, 2011).

Bakos, Susan Crain. *The Sex Bible for Women: The Complete Guide to Understanding Your Body, Being a Great Lover, and Getting the Pleasure You Want*. Beverly, MA: Quiver, 2008.

Bass, Ellen, and Laura Davis. *The Courage to Heal: A Guide for Women Survivors of Child Sexual Abuse*. 3rd ed. New York: Harper, 1994.

Bean, Joseph W. *Flogging*. Emeryville, CA: Greenery, 2000.

Berman, Jennifer, Laura Berman, and Elisabeth Bumiller. *For Women Only: A Revolutionary Guide to Overcoming Sexual Dysfunction and Reclaiming Your Sex Life*. New York: Henry Holt and Co., 2001.

Berman, Laura. *Real Sex for Real Women: Intimacy, Pleasure & Sexual Well-Being*. New York: DK Pub., 2008.

Briggs, Laura. "The Race of Hysteria: 'Overcivilization' and the 'Savage' in Late Nineteenth-Century Obstetrics and Gynecology." *American Quarterly* 52, no. 2 (2000): 246–73.

Brown, Patricia Leigh, and Carol Pogash. "The Pleasure Principle." *New York Times*, March 15, 2009.

Carrellas, Barbara. *Urban Tantra: Sacred Sex for the Twenty-First Century.* Berkeley, CA: Celestial Arts, 2007.

Chalker, Rebecca. *The Clitoral Truth: The Secret World at Your Fingertips.* New York: Seven Stories, 2002.

Christensen, Birgitte, Morton Grønbæk, and Christian Graugaard. "Associations of Unhealthy Lifestyle Factors with Sexual Inactivity and Sexual Dysfunctions in Denmark." *Journal of Sexual Medicine* 8, no. 7 (2011): 1903–16.

Dutton, Judy. *Secrets from the Sex Lab: From First Kiss to Last Gasp—How You Can Be Better in Bed.* New York: Broadway, 2009.

Easton, Dossie, and Janet W. Hardy. *Radical Ecstasy: SM Journeys to Transcendence.* Oakland, CA: Greenery, 2004.

Easton, Dossie, and Janet W. Hardy. *The Ethical Slut: A Practical Guide to Polyamory, Open Relationships & Other Adventures.* Berkeley, CA: Celestial Arts, 2009.

Fausto-Sterling, Anne. *Sexing the Body: Gender Politics and the Construction of Sexuality.* New York: Basic, 2000.

Ferber, Abby L., Kimberly Holcomb, and Tre Wentling. *Sex, Gender, and Sexuality: The New Basics—an Anthology.* New York: Oxford University Press, 2009.

FetishDiva, Midori, Linda Santiman, and Steve Diet Goedde. *Wild Side Sex: The Book of Kink—Educational, Sensual, and Entertaining Essays.* Los Angeles: Daedalus, 2005.

Fisher, Helen E. *Why We Love: The Nature and Chemistry of Romantic Love.* New York: Henry Holt and Co., 2005.

Galinsky, Adena M., and Freya L. Sonenstein. "The Association Between Developmental Assets and Sexual Enjoyment Among Emerging Adults." *Journal of Adolescent Health* 48, no. 6 (2011): 610–15.

Groneman, Carol. *Nymphomania: A History.* New York: W. W. Norton, 2000.

Hartley, Nina, and I. S. Levine. *Nina Hartley's Guide to Total Sex.* New York: Avery, 2006.

Herbenick, Debby. *Because It Feels Good: A Woman's Guide to Sexual Pleasure and Satisfaction.* New York: Rodale Inc., 2009.

Herbenick, Debra, Michael Reece, Stephanie Sanders, Brian Dodge, Annahita Ghassemi, and J. Dennis Fortenberry. "Prevalence and Characteristics of Vibrator Use by Women in the United States: Results from a Nationally Representative Study." *Journal of Sexual Medicine* 6, no. 7 (2009): 1857–66.

Herbenick, Debra. "The Development and Validation of a Scale to Measure Attitudes Toward Women's Genitals." *International Journal of Sexual Health* 21, no. 3 (2009): 153–66.

Hughes, Susan M., Marissa A. Harrison, and Gordon G. Gallup. "Sex Differences in Romantic Kissing Among College Students: An Evolutionary Perspective." *Evolutionary Psychology* 5, no. 3 (2007): 612–31.

Kinetz, Erika. "Is Hysteria Real? Brain Images Say Yes." *New York Times,* September 26, 2006.

Komisaruk, Barry R., Carlos Beyer, and Beverly Whipple. *The Science of Orgasm.* Baltimore: Johns Hopkins University Press, 2006.

Ladas, Alice Kahn, Beverly Whipple, and John D. Perry. *The G Spot: And Other Discoveries About Human Sexuality.* New York: Henry Holt and Co., 2005.

Laqueur, Thomas Walter. *Making Sex: Body and Gender from the Greeks to Freud.* Cambridge, MA: Harvard University Press, 1992.

Laqueur, Thomas Walter. *Solitary Sex: A Cultural History of Masturbation.* New York: Zone, 2003.

Maines, Rachel. *The Technology of Orgasm: "Hysteria," the Vibrator, and Women's Sexual Satisfaction.* Baltimore, MD: Johns Hopkins University Press, 2001.

Margolis, Jonathan. *O: The Intimate History of the Orgasm.* New York: Grove, 2004.

Morin, Jack. *The Erotic Mind: Unlocking the Inner Sources of Sexual Passion and Fulfillment.* New York: HarperCollins, 1995.

Nestle, Joan, Clare Howell, and Riki Anne Wilchins. *GenderQueer: Voices from Beyond the Sexual Binary*. Los Angeles: Alyson, 2002.

Newman, Felice. *The Whole Lesbian Sex Book: A Passionate Guide for All of Us*. San Francisco: Cleis, 2004.

Odem, Mary E. *Delinquent Daughters: Protecting and Policing Adolescent Female Sexuality in the United States, 1885–1920*. Chapel Hill, NC: University of North Carolina Press, 1995.

Parker-Pope, Tara. *For Better: The Science of a Good Marriage*. New York: Dutton, 2010.

Queen, Carol. *Exhibitionism for the Shy: Show Off, Dress Up, and Talk Hot*. San Francisco: Down There, 1995.

Reece, Michael, Debra Herbenick, Stephanie A. Sanders, Brian Dodge, Annahita Ghassemi, and J. Dennis Fortenberry. "Prevalence and Characteristics of Vibrator Use by Men in the United States." *Journal of Sexual Medicine* 6, no. 7 (2009): 1867–74.

Roach, Mary. *Bonk: The Curious Coupling of Science and Sex*. New York: W. W. Norton, 2008.

"Sexual Activity Reported in Dreams of Men and Women." *Science Daily: News & Articles in Science, Health, Environment & Technology*. www.sciencedaily.com/releases/2007/06/070614085118.htm (accessed June 26, 2011).

Solot, Dorian, and Marshall Miller. *I [Heart] Female Orgasm: An Extraordinary Orgasm Guide*. Cambridge, MA: Da Capo Press, 2007.

Stein, Rob. "The Differences in Gender—Sealed with a Kiss." *Washington Post*, February 11, 2008.

"Study: Sexual Insecurity Leads to Cheating." *YourTango*, June 21, 2011. www.yourtango.com/201178937/study-sexual-insecurity-leads-cheating (accessed June 25, 2011).

Taormino, Tristan. *Opening Up: A Guide to Creating and Sustaining Open Relationships*. San Francisco: Cleis, 2008.

Taylor, Timothy. *The Prehistory of Sex: Four Million Years of Human Sexual Culture*. New York: Bantam, 1996.

The-Clitoris.com. www.the-clitoris.com. (accessed June 26, 2011).

The-Penis.com. www.the-penis.com. (accessed June 26, 2011).

Tisdale, Sallie. *Talk Dirty to Me: An Intimate Philosophy of Sex.* New York: Anchor, 1995.

"Uncovering the Truth: Why Women 'Fake It.'" *LiveScience,* June 6, 2011. www.livescience.com/14451-fear-intimacy-faking-orgasm.html (accessed June 26, 2011).

"What's the Secret of Hot Sex? Science Weighs In." *CBS News,* June 15, 2011. www.cbsnews.com/8301-504763_162-20071130-10391704 .html (accessed June 25, 2011).

ACKNOWLEDGMENTS

I WANT TO ACKNOWLEDGE some of the writers whose work has helped shape my thinking about sex: Barbara Carrellas, Kate Bornstein, Carol Queen, Midori, Tristan Taormino, Dossie Easton, Janet Hardy, Annie Sprinkle and Beth Stevens, Julia Serano, Helen Boyd, Patrick Califia, Gayle Rubin, Ducky DooLittle. Thanks to Don Weise for helping shape the idea for this book, and for his interest in and smart approach to books on sexuality. Thanks to Metis Black of Tantus Inc. and Jack Lamon of Come As You Are for providing inspiration and reliable, smart information about sexuality.

Thanks to my editor, Brooke Warner, for saving this project when its original publisher failed. I appreciate her patience and guidance. Thanks to friends in New York and Philadelphia who listened, let me bounce ideas off them, and provided inspiration through great conversations about sex and gender. Special thanks to my partner, Emma Crandall, who has been my cheerleader, my champion, and a source of unwavering support. She was patient, loving, attentive, and gracious throughout the process of writing this book. I literally could not have written it without her.

ABOUT THE AUTHOR

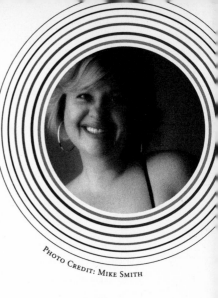

DIANA CAGE is a former editor of the influential lesbian sex magazine *On Our Backs* and former host of Sirius XM's *The Diana Cage Show*. Her eight previous books include *Box Lunch, Girl Meets Girl, Threeways,* and *The On Our Backs Guide to Lesbian Sex.* Diana holds an MFA from San Francisco State University and teaches Women's Sexualities at Brooklyn College. She has spoken about sexuality and gender at universities around the country.

SELECTED TITLES FROM SEAL PRESS

For more than thirty years, Seal Press has published groundbreaking books. By women. For women.

Getting Off: A Woman's Guide to Masturbation, by Jamye Waxman, illustrations by Molly Crabapple. $15.95, 978-1-58005-219-1. Empowering and female-positive, this is a comprehensive guide for women on the history and mechanics of the oldest and most common sexual practice.

Sexual Intimacy for Women: A Guide for Same-Sex Couples, by Glenda Corwin, Ph.D. $16.95, 978-1-58005-303-7. In this prescriptive and poignant book, Glenda Corwin, PhD, helps female couples overcome obstacles to sexual intimacy through her examination of the emotional, physical, and psychological aspects of same-sex relationships.

What You Really Really Want: The Smart Girl's Shame-Free Guide to Sex and Safety, by Jaclyn Friedman. $17.00, 978-1-58005-344-0. An educational and interactive guide that gives young women the tools they need to decipher the modern world's confusing, hypersexualized landscape and define their own sexual identity.

Sexier Sex: Lessons from the Brave New Sexual Frontier, by Regina Lynn. $14.95, 978-1-58005-231-3. A fun, provocative guide to discovering your sexuality and getting more pleasure from your sensual life.

Curvy Girls: Erotica for Women, edited by Rachel Kramer Bussel. $18.00, 978-1-58005-408-9. A voluptuously erotic collection showcasing the sensuality of larger women in all their curvy glory, from the sexiness of big butts and plus-size corsets to the irresistible allure of pregnant bellies.

Affection: An Erotic Memoir, by Krissy Kneen. $16.95, 978-1-58005-342-6. A powerful, explicit, and sexy account of an extraordinarily sensual woman's experiences with sex, from adolescence to adulthood, and an examination of how her sense of self shapes and is shaped by those experiences.

Find Seal Press Online
www.SealPress.com
www.Facebook.com/SealPress
Twitter: @SealPress